"Dr. Fountain is interested in th  person. *God, Medicine, and Mi* when spirituality has re-entere practice through the side door of an interest in mind-body medicine. Dr. Fountain sees patients as the trinity they are: souls, inhabiting bodies who have spirits. From the viewpoint of the patient as well as of the physician-healer, spiritual resources available to both patients and physicians are deeply explored and clarified in a manner that brings hope to the patient as well as the physician."
—*C. Everett Koop, M.D., Sc.D.*, senior scholar, C. Everett Koop Institute at Dartmouth; surgeon general, 1981–1989

"The work of Daniel Fountain is an amazing story that proves that more things are wrought through prayer than this world can possibly imagine. This missionary doctor explains how spiritual disciplines can bring hope and help to those who suffer from even the most dreaded disease of our time, and he backs up his claims with case studies."
—*Tony Campolo, Ph.D.*, Eastern College, St. Davids, Pennsylvania

"Science is finding out what Christians have known for a long time—spirituality has an impact on health. With the wisdom of the Great Physician, Dr. Fountain shares insights from decades of practice that will warm your heart and change your life. This book is great medicine for body and soul."
—*David Stevens, M.D.*, executive director of the Christian Medical and Dental Society

"I was deeply blessed and stretched in mind and heart while reading—literally devouring—Dr. Daniel

Fountain's provocative, helpful book. I hope a host of thoughtful laypeople as well as those in the medical community will read Dr. Fountain's teaching and take it to heart. This is not theory. The first-hand stories of people who have been healed—spiritually, physically, and emotionally—powerfully illustrate all that Dr. Fountain is teaching us. Out of Dr. Fountain's distinguished, pioneering—and deeply Christian—thirty-five years of medical practice in central Africa, as well as his profound grasp of Scripture, we are given an understanding of what 'holistic medicine' is all about."
—*Dr. Roger L. Fredrikson,* professor, pastor, and author

"No person is better qualified to speak authoritatively about the issues of spirituality in health and healing than Dr. Dan Fountain. From his unique vantage point as a medical missionary he has first-hand experience with total dependence on God when dealing with imponderables in health. Through his personal faith in Christ, careful reflections, submission to scriptural authority, and ability to listen to God, he has lifted whole-person medicine to a higher stage of development. Spiritual healing is not an 'alternative therapy' but, rather, integral in all therapies for illness, leading to wholeness of spirit, mind, emotions, relationships, and body."
—*David S. Topazian, DDS, MBA,* President of Project MedSend

GOD,
MEDICINE
& MIRACLES

Isaiah 53 The Lord is our Healer
Dan Fountain

The Spiritual Factor in Healing

Daniel E. Fountain, M.D.

SHAW

WATERBROOK
P R E S S

God, Medicine, and Miracles
A SHAW BOOK
PUBLISHED BY WATERBROOK PRESS
2375 Telstar Drive, Suite 160
Colorado Springs, CO 80920
A division of Random House, Inc.

ISBN: 0-87788-321-1

Edited by Elisa Fryling and Vinita Hampton Wright
Cover design by Thomas Leo
Cover photo © 1990, VCG/FPG International LLC

Library of Congress Cataloging-in-Publication Data

Fountain, Daniel E.
    God, medicine, and miracles / Daniel E. Fountain.
        p. cm.
    Includes bibliographical references.
    ISBN 0-87788-321-1 (pbk.)
        1. Medicine—Religious aspects—Christianity.   2. Healing—Religious aspects—Christianity.   I. Title.
    BT732.F68   1999
    261.5'61—dc21   99-24093
                                        CIP

Printed in the United States of America

05   04   03   02

10   9   8   7   6   5   4   3

To John, Deborah, Roger, Nellie, Patrice, and Michael, who have been healed by Jesus Christ, and to the multitude of my sisters and brothers who need healing.

"He healed our diseases and made us well."
Matthew 8:17 (CEV)

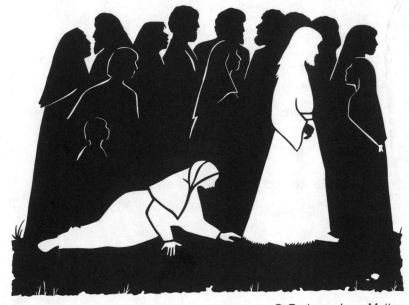

© Barbara Jean Mattes

Contents

Foreword

Books on healing and faith are not new. Many have been written by physicians. O. Carl Simonton, Herbert Benson, and Bernie Siegel come to mind. These and many other authors have dared to tackle this subject because they all have experienced a correlation between their patients' faith and the state of their health. Some consider the bridge between faith and health purely psychological. For some, the idea of *faith* is vague enough to include every sort of religious belief: any faith will do. What counts, some insist, is a positive, hopeful, and confident mental attitude—however you come by it.

But these books and others like them, while they do challenge some very stubborn and time-worn materialistic prejudices, have usually left the issue of spiritual reality alone. For some, faith is no more than believing that somehow things will be better, so you can have hope and work at getting well. Whether the thing believed in truly exists is left unmentioned. But there is an important issue here. If I am to believe something, I must think it is true, real, and really "there."

The issue, briefly stated, is this: Does a realm of reality exist that is important to human health and is not material? Not psychological? Not reducible to biochemical explanation? In short, is there a transcendent God and does a relationship with God through Jesus Christ contribute something to healing—additional to chemical and physical variables? To put the question another way, given that faith heals, does it make any difference which faith we are talking about?

Although voluminous research has been published showing the healing power of faith, I am not aware of research demonstrating that specifically *Christian* faith possesses superior efficacy. That faith can produce miracles has never been considered a unique capacity of Christianity alone. The magicians of Egypt evidently replicated the miracles produced by Moses. And if any religion can be shown to aid its adherents in developing psychologically effective attitudes, Christians ought to have no difficulty accepting the phenomenon even if they reject the religion. After all, God makes his rain fall on everybody, even if their religion is untrue.

Although I do not know of any controlled research proving that it is so, I nevertheless believe that the truth will, in the long run, prove to deploy more healing power than having ever-so-much faith in that which is not the truth. I am convinced therefore that specifically *Christian* faith will be shown to contribute superior efficacy.

This is not just another book about faith and healing. Rather, it is about specifically *Christian* faith and how that faith contributes to human wholeness. Belief that includes obedience to the teachings of Christ and the freeing power of the Holy Spirit can and does result in healing beyond that produced by medicine, surgery, and psychology. Dr. Dan Fountain here tells of his own experience with clinical events that answer, to his satisfaction, the question of the healing power of faith, prayer, and obedience to the Word of God.

When I first received a letter from Dr. Fountain, I had never met him. That letter and subsequent correspondence meant the start of an important new journey for me. As a clinical psychologist I already knew the power of truth for the healing of *psychological* disorders. But here was a physician in Zaire (now the Congo) who described a brilliant, new Spirit-inspired AIDS treatment program he and his staff were using at the Vanga Hospital in Kinshasa, Zaire. The AIDS epidemic had ravaged many African countries while doctors there often did not have AIDS medications at their disposal. But Dr. Fountain believed that, lacking the resources to medicate his patients, he could help them treat themselves with positive truth. And since he had come across several books I had written on psychological healing by the truth as it is in Jesus, he thought we ought to converse.

Fountain's daring venture into *positive truth treatment* has brought fresh life and hope to people who might, otherwise, have been left to believe nothing could save them—a message all too often given to sick people the world over, including persons with AIDS, cancer, and heart disease in those countries like the United States where there are drugs aplenty.

Teaching and wise counseling by the hospital's pastoral staff, such as this book describes, along with the patient's deep commitment to Christ and thorough instruction in the healing power of the blood of Christ in the deep mind, would have power to touch the patient's violated immune system and improve its functioning. Fountain is not talking only about miraculous cures, but also and especially about the completely normal, built-in fact that a mind filled with God's truth and saturated with the Word and Spirit of Christ can effect a more healthy body. In Fountain's own words in personal correspondence,

> Medical science is vigorously attacking the [HIV] virus, assuming that victory over the virus will solve the problem . . . [this] will

not, of course, even touch the multitude of problems involved in the complex etiology of HIV infection. We . . . are working on the other side of the problem, with the immune system, trying through psycho-social-spiritual means to strengthen the immune system so it can better cope with the infection. Can it ever be sufficiently strengthened to eliminate the infection? As Paul wrote to the Colossians: "Christ is the key that opens all the hidden treasures of God's wisdom and knowledge." (Colossians 2:3)

I was thunderstruck! Would it be possible to find people who had been helped toward better health and even healed of seemingly incurable illnesses by learning how to tell themselves positive, even spiritual truth? Could such fresh, upbeat, optimistic truth really recharge weakened immune systems? I did not think Christian theologians had yet done relevant work on this issue. Had scientists any hard data? Had any other doctors actually tried programs similar to Dan Fountain's program working with, say, cancer patients, heart patients, AIDS patients?

A significant fact seemed to be widely ignored. *Some people recover from the worst illnesses no matter how doom-laden the statistics might be!* But an important question was rarely being asked. *Why? Why did those who were supposed to die* not *die? Why did those who were supposed to become ill* not *become ill?*

Shortly after Fountain and I began to correspond, the Associated Press carried the news that Dr. Stephen Ostroff, of the U.S. Center for Disease Control, had noted the supreme importance of these question for understanding the Ebola epidemic then raging in Africa. Dr. Ostroff said, "Each of the individuals who survive [Ebola] are very valuable. Why? Because they may help us understand how to survive this virulent virus. Medicine, psychology, and religion must study the people who *don't* get sick. This is a time in history when precisely that study is taking place on a scale never before imagined."

As I read Dr. Ostroff's words, something stirred in my heart. It seemed to me that Ostroff's question was a crucial one and that the patient's spirit might very well be part of the answer to it. Why *do* some people survive fatal illnesses? Of course! We would expect the spirit filled with the Spirit of Truth to make a difference, not simply in a person's after-death destination, but in *everything,* including the immune system and the power to resist and overcome illness.

If this expectation is correct, then a mind filled with the truth of God would result in exactly what the Scriptures promise: strength, not only supernatural, miraculous strength (although God certainly does miracles even today), not merely spiritual and mental strength, but physical strength! Deep in my spirit, I was convinced that *telling yourself heartening, encouraging truth has the power to help you move toward physical wholeness.*

For some time now, science, including medical science, has been taught, has learned, and all too often has practiced as if a person had no spirit, as if there were no God, and as if such issues as spirit and God have no relevance in the practice of medicine. Once, the ideal clinical practice was thought to be purely scientific. And in this framework *scientific* meant construing reality as *nothing but* matter. The habit of *reductionism* makes things simple by pretending that everything comes down to matter and energy.

So "this earth with its store of wonders untold" is reduced to nothing more than a ball of dirt hanging out there in the dark, cold, impersonal universe like a speck of dust in a bell jar. And the human being is likewise reduced to no more than a fleck of organic scum of infinitesimal significance in the great scheme of things. So the doctor was taught to see illness, physical and mental, as no more than the malfunctioning of chemicals, and the distortion of structures. It follows that if your spirit is crushed, take a pill. If your heart is broken, change your diet. If you feel guilty, go on vacation. If you are anxious, try a tranquilizer. If you have cancer, all we can do is cut it out, medicate, irradiate, or give up.

This book takes you into a fascinatingly rich new realm of medical practice. One where the material is not neglected, but seen as properly subordinated to the spiritual, and finding well-being and health in that submission and subordination. The practical working out of this new, multifaceted kind of medical practice Dan Fountain spells out in story after story: Roger, who was dying of liver disease before obedience to the truth of God led to a rapid recovery; John, whose fatal illness was reversed when he was taught that the truth of Jesus was mightier than an uncle's curse; Deborah, whose healing came as, by faith and by the Word of God, she heard Jesus call her "daughter," and more.

These pages hold many wonderful gifts for the reader. Among them is hope—hope for the sick and those who care for them, including clinicians—hope for the well against a time of illness in the future.

William Backus, Ph.D., S.T.M.

Words of Thanks

Many of God's best gifts come to us through other people. This book is no exception. Much of what I have learned about health, illness, and healing, God has brought to me through many mentors. I want to acknowledge them here.

Countless sick persons have shown me that illness penetrates deeper than the flesh. Many of these people have been willing to expose their soul to me in the hope that, together, we could find a healing balm. In spite of my often impetuous manner and my urge to rush from one sick person to another, these people have constrained me to seek remedies more powerful than pills, antiseptics, or an array of surgical instruments. Slowly I have learned that I cannot touch the soul and spirit of a sick person with latex gloves. Nor can I touch them while hiding behind a white coat. To these wonderful people, many of whom have found healing, I owe an immense debt of gratitude.

A wonderful family of colleagues has accompanied me on this journey of learning from the Great Physician. Outstanding among them is Mrs. Felicity Matala, an African woman to whom God has given many gifts. Her understanding of deep truths in the Bible, her discernment of the real ills of hurting people, and her compassionate and gentle way of bringing healing resources to these people have unlocked many mysteries of healing. Together we have seen the pervasive and destructive effects of illness on the human spirit. We have also discovered the marvelous power of faith in

God to restore soul, spirit, and body.

A dedicated team of fellow physicians, some of them African, others German, Swiss, and North American, has been part of this learning process. Many of the questions and ideas in this book came as we have consulted together, made rounds in the wards, or gathered to discuss God's Word and, at the same time, human illness and particular diseases. Members of the nursing and technical support staff and the administrative personnel of our hospital in the Congo have contributed much to a deeper grasp of what is involved in healing.

I have drawn on the wisdom of wise mentors of the past. Sir William Osler, Dr. Paul Tournier, Dr. Paul Brand, and professors and fellow learners from university and medical training years have implanted in my mind solid principles of the wholeness of life. They have insisted that I pay attention to spiritual issues, to personal relationships, and to the lifestyle of sick persons. They have showed me the crucial importance of listening carefully to what sick persons are really trying to tell me.

The editorial staff at Harold Shaw Publishers has given invaluable counsel and encouragement. Right from the beginning, it was clear to my spirit as well as to my mind that their principal interest was not just to publish another book. They have caught the vision of this book—that of caring for the whole person—and, like me, want to make it available to the hurting people who need it and also to those who are caregivers. They have worked tirelessly with me to help clarify and refine the message so that it can speak to hearts as well as to minds.

My own family has shared in this with me from the beginning. For Miriam, this has been her life as well as mine. We have wrestled together with perplexing issues, fought against the common enemies of pestilence, ignorance, and many of the evils that seek to destroy human lives. We have wept together as we have lost a few skirmishes. But she has helped me keep alive the faith that God wills life and health, and that the battles we fight are his battles. Together with God we have participated in many victories.

Our children and now our grandchildren have taken part in this vision as well. I rejoice in this because it is to them, as well as to a host of fellow healers, that I pass the baton.

Introduction

To get sick is to be human; illness touches everyone in one way or another. When we get sick, it is only natural that we want to get well. We want to get rid of the pain, fever, weakness, or whatever the discomfort may be. If we are really sick, we go to someone we believe can help us get well. But do we always find the help we need?

Sickness, Healing, and the Whole Person

The medical profession has a major problem—I can say this because I am a physician. We focus too much on the disease and on the particular part of the body that appears to be sick. We pay too little attention to the person who is sick and how he or she is trying to cope with the illness.

When I was a small boy, I developed tuberculosis. The pediatrician told my parents that it was in the right upper lobe of my lungs and in lymph glands in my chest and neck. I did not realize until years later that I—not just one lobe of my lungs and a few lymph glands—had been sick.

During my surgical residency I assisted the chief resident at the Veterans Administration Hospital in removing two-thirds of the stomach of a thirty-year-old veteran. We had worked with him unsuccessfully for months to convince him to stop drinking. When his stomach ulcer bled profusely, we were forced to operate to save his life. Three days later, as we examined him on rounds, he asked my chief, "Doctor, when can I start drinking again?" We had saved his life by removing the sick part of his stomach, but we had failed to heal him.

Healing has to do with soul and spirit as well as with the body. Deep inside, we sense this, yet we health professionals have neglected this aspect of healing for too long. When you come to us, you tell us where you hurt and how you feel. But seldom do we inquire about how you live or what your deep worries, fears, and stresses are. Part of the problem is that we simply don't have the time. So you—as a whole person—go away underevaluated and inadequately helped.

In the book of Isaiah we find a very significant proverb: "The bed is too short to stretch out on, the blanket too narrow to wrap around you" (Isaiah 28:20, NIV). Isaiah could not have made a more apt analysis about modern medicine and our health care system. Medical science has devised a marvelous bed for sick persons, but it is too short. Only your body can fit into it; there is no room for your soul or spirit. Psychology has knitted a cozy blanket, but it is too narrow. It does not cover your spirit.

As persons we are spiritual beings; we are social beings as well. Medical science does wonders with the physical, and psychology can do much with the psychological. But the healing of the soul and the spirit, the reestablishing of right relationships with others, and the restoration of the whole person—these require something more.

I believe God has made this world and all that is in it, including us. I believe that God is good, that he made everything good, and that his plan for us is good. That plan includes health, life, and joy. Reality, however, is different. We are frequently ill, life often loses its meaning and purpose, and we will never arrive at complete wholeness in this world. So where are God and his goodness and love in all of this? Can we find help from God, and hope for healing and health?

We read in the Bible that God came into our world as Jesus of Nazareth. Jesus healed people during his life on earth. Does he still heal sick persons today as he did two thousand years ago? I believe he does, although I do not pretend to have answers to all of the many questions this raises. As I have struggled with these questions and with who we are as persons, I have learned something that may be of value to you in sickness and in health, or when you are caring for someone else who is ill.

God wants us to study the world he has created, and he has given us the intelligence to do so. Our study includes the sciences, and these include medicine and psychology in their many branches. These sciences have gone far to help us when we are ill. Yet something more is needed, or rather, Someone more.

The Bible says that Jesus is the Savior. Our modern languages do not do justice to the ancient Hebrew and Greek words that we translate as savior. The Hebrew word "Yeshua" and the Greek word "Sotera" mean both savior and healer. The two concepts are included in both the Hebrew and Greek words. *This means that healing is a part of salvation.* "Yeshua," or "salvation," means deliverance, health, healing, salvation, or saving health. The full meaning of salvation is to be made whole, to be saved from sin, sorrow, and sickness. Jesus is our Healer as well as our Savior. For this reason he has been called the Great Physician.

Are you suffering from an illness that persists in spite of what you and medical science have been able to do? Are there pains in your body or troubles in your mind or spirit that will not go away? Is there any hope for relief, for a return to health, and for moving toward a fuller life and joy?

Perhaps you have loved ones who are ill, handicapped, or in great distress. You have cared for them, counseled them, prayed for them, and taken them to this doctor and to that clinic, all to no avail. Can anything more be done?

God Has Provided Resources for Us

God has made available to us many resources to protect our health and to help us recover from illness. Some of these resources are within us—the body's built-in systems and the inner life of our emotions and choices. We will be discussing these resources in some detail. Medical science provides additional resources for both mind and body. We also have available to us another potent therapeutic resource: faith, specifically faith in Jesus Christ.

Perhaps you know little, or nothing at all, about God or Jesus Christ, but you are still interested in this book's content. That's all right. If you are ill, and your own resources plus all that health science and professionals have done for you have been insufficient to restore you to health and wholeness, this book may help you. It may help you see more fully who *you* really are. You will see the wonderful resources God has put within us to keep us healthy, how things go wrong that make us ill, and what we can do about them. Spiritual resources can have physiological benefits, and faith is a major factor in health and in healing.

In this book we will look at the following questions:

1. How do our emotions, feelings, and beliefs—our inner self—affect our health?

2. When illness comes, how can we moblize mental, emotional, and spiritual resources to help our bodies cope?

3. What can faith in Jesus Christ, together with the healing sciences, do to help us when we are ill?

I have come at these questions from both sides. I have lain for long months in bed. I have been on the operating table looking up. I have seen death peering through the window and have hoped it would go away. I have struggled against pain, weakness, and the frustration of having a spirit that is willing but flesh that is weak.

During much of my life I have also sat at the bedside of others who suffer. I have looked down on many persons on the operating table and asked God to help me do what would facilitate their healing. I have listened to the stories of many sick persons and tried to respond in ways that encouraged them in their journey toward health. In all of this I have consulted textbooks of medicine as well as the Great Physician. Over the years, in many different ways, God and medical science have been teaching me about healing, and I continue to be a learner. In these pages you will find a bit of what I have learned from God. It is, as it were, only the "edges of his ways," for the full extent of his ways are past finding out (Romans 11:33, KJV).

1

Does the Doctor Know Who You Are?

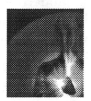

Are you a person, or are you simply a bunch of separate organs held together by connective tissue? Are you an isolated individual, or are you a member of a family, a community, and a network of friends and colleagues? Are you just a highly complex mass of carbohydrates and amino and fatty acids that can somehow think, or are you a being who is in relationship with other spiritual powers in the universe?

When you go to your physician, how do you want him or her to look at you? As a possible case of gall stones? As a probable coronary patient? Or do you hope that physician will see you as a person in which something has gone wrong?

A Whole Person?

Western culture has radically altered our concept of human beings. Our scientific achievements have led us to believe that, by dissection and molecular biology, we can understand all that is important about ourselves. Our popular culture and even many of our religious beliefs and practices have emphasized the individual and neglected the impact that relationships have on us. In our reverence for reason we have often assumed that there is nothing in life or in nature that our minds will not eventually be able to understand and thus manipulate.

All of this has greatly affected our approach to health and to illness. Modern medicine has become mechanical, technical, and compartmentalized. When you are ill, physicians focus on trying to find out what has gone wrong and how it can be fixed. We note your name and personal information primarily in order to fill out your medical and insurance forms.

During my third year in medical school, I spent some months in the out-patient clinics. I began the rotation in the general medicine clinic. A middle-aged woman came complaining of long-standing low back pain. The intern and I presumed she had an orthopedic problem, and we referred her to that clinic. A few days later she was sent back to us with a note stating that all examinations of her low back, bones, and joints indicated no bone or joint disease.

We referred her to the gynecological clinic, but she soon returned with a note from them stating that they could find no signs of disease in her pelvic organs. The urology clinic was next, and after extensive laboratory and radiographic examinations, no disease was found in her kidneys or urinary tract. Finally, she went to the neurology clinic, where nothing unusual was discovered.

When this woman returned to us, three things were evident. Her pain was unchanged, her money was gone, and we had failed to help her. She left the clinic, and we never saw her again. Only later did I remember that none of us had sat down with her to talk about her life and how her illness had developed. We were trying to treat her pain but had failed to recognize her as a person.

A few weeks later, however, in the internal medicine clinic, I did much better. I was excited when I discovered rales (fine crackling sounds) in the lung bases of a sixty-something woman who was complaining of shortness of breath. She also had swelling of her ankles and lower legs. It was evident that she was in mild heart failure and that we could help her. Under the resident's supervision, I prescribed digoxin, a stimulant of the heart muscles, and a diuretic medicine, and a week later she was much improved. I then talked to her about long-term care, including a low-salt diet, mild exercise, and regular return visits to the clinic.

This lady went home satisfied, and I felt fulfilled. Here was a therapeutic triumph. However, a week later, I could not remember her name or where she lived. Was she married? I had not asked her. How was her life at home with her family, and with her friends? Could she have had stress problems that were adding to the work of her heart? I never inquired. It did not occur to me until much later that I had treated, not a woman, but a cardiac muscle.

The Biomedical Model

This is what we call the biomedical model of medical care. We health professionals are trained to consider the person as a biological and physical being. Something biological goes wrong with the physical body that requires a medical intervention. We understand a lot about the mechanisms that keep us alive and well—our digestion, our respiration, our circulation, and other "-ations" that are more intimate. We consider disease to be a breakdown in one or more of these mechanisms and that our role is to repair what has gotten out of order. But where is the person in this model?

We do have a lot of mechanisms going on inside of us, and lots of things can go wrong with them. However, as persons we are so much more than "mechanisms." We think, we feel, we struggle, and we hope. We relate to other people, and in these relationships we often find joy and satisfaction, and sometimes frustration and anger.

Unfortunately it is taking health professionals far too long to realize that the frustration and anger we sometimes feel can upset some of those biological mechanisms. At the same time, the joy, laughter, and fulfillment we find with family or friends can often restore many ill-functioning mechanisms better than can our fancy medicines and complicated technology. These were matters I did not learn in my training.

My Personal Journey with Illness

One of the most helpful experiences that we physicians can have is to be ill ourselves. I have learned much during numerous episodes of illness—not as much about biomedical matters as about caring for the whole person. That learning process began long before I studied medicine. It began when I was seven years old, the day that a wise pediatrician looked at my chest X-ray and announced to my mother and father, "Your Danny has tuberculosis."

This word struck fear into the hearts of my parents, for that was in 1937, ten years before the antibiotic era began. Tuberculosis was still a major killer, especially of young children. The "triple therapy" at that time was not three drugs; it consisted of bed rest, good food, and lots of sunshine. The prescription for me was a year of bed rest followed by at least three years of limited activity. The doctor gave us a choice: putting me in a well-equipped sanatorium one hundred and fifty miles away and staffed by trained personnel, or letting me stay in bed at home. For my parents, there was no decision: I would stay at home.

For a hyperactive boy like me, the prospect of being in bed for a year was depressing to say the least. Although my parents were firm in enforcing the prescription, they compensated for it by much tender loving care. I soon learned something important. A disease could restrict my bodily activity, but it did not need to inhibit my mind, my spirit, or my creativity. Books became my companions. The overturned bed table was transformed into a ship in which I could sail the seven seas. I discovered that Jesus was my friend, and we would talk for hours. We crossed the Sea of Galilee, tramped through forests, and climbed high mountains together. As I read his book, the Bible, I collected nuggets of wisdom that have guided me ever since. Within a month my mind, my heart, and my spirit were healed. I believe this sped up the healing of my lungs and the lymph nodes in my chest.

Many years later, as I analyzed this illness that had occurred during a very formative stage in my life, and as I realized what had happened to me, many questions came to mind. Was I simply cured of tuberculosis, or did I become whole? Was it just my lungs that had recovered, or had my whole self changed for the better? I was indeed cured of tuberculosis, but how? The white blood cells in my lungs and lymph nodes had somehow gobbled up the tuberculosis bacilli, but what else had happened to make me well?

It became clear to me that the year 1937–1938 had been a special year for me. I had learned much: skills in reading and writing, patience in waiting, creativity in imagination, and visions of eventually doing something about illness and disease to make life better for other people. Friends came to visit. My second-grade teacher sent home schoolwork each day, and I was able to keep up my studies. I also received much love and care from my parents; they were true caregivers. Regular visits to the pediatrician gave additional assurance that I was on the right track.

In retrospect, I saw that my mind and spirit had grown much during that year. This came not in spite of the disease, but largely because of it and with the help of family and friends. Did all of this somehow help my lungs and lymph nodes in their battle against the infection? I began to see that what happened to me as a whole person strongly influenced and facilitated my recovery from the disease.

My Medical Training

When I entered medical school at the University of Rochester years later, I was challenged and delighted by the marvels of medical science. The magnificent anatomy of the body, the stupendous complexities of the functioning of the various organs, and the intricate associations between them—all of this fascinated me.

At the same time, I continued reading my Bible and learning about Jesus. I read about healing in the Bible and saw examples of this in the ministry of Christ. Much of it seemed to go beyond medicine, at least beyond what I was learning of medical science. What did Jesus mean when he said to a sick person, "Your faith has made you whole"? Were all the healings Jesus accomplished actual miracles? Or, in some instances at least, did he use principles and methods that are available to us now?

I began to wonder how to put medicine and faith together. Unfortunately, there was no one to help me, for these two areas of life were carefully kept separate. Medical science excludes faith because science cannot measure it. (Science can't disprove faith, either.) But what I learned in church did not deal with scientific knowledge or technology. I discovered that trying to examine miracles from a scientific point of view was often regarded as denying the power of God. But doesn't God have anything to do with science? It would seem so, since science studies what God has made and done.

I struggled to understand how Jesus fit into this picture. I remember clearly how, as a young intern, I was standing in the nursing station of the acute psychiatric ward in the Philadelphia General Hospital. I could look down both corridors through the large glass windows. I knew who was in every bed in each room. I was watching an older Irishman in the manic phase of a manic-depressive disorder dancing a jig around a tall, stately African-American man standing immobile in a catatonic pose in the middle of the corridor. Each was oblivious of the other. A burning question in my heart rose heavenward. *Lord, if you could spend ten minutes in this ward, you could heal all forty of these suffering people. Can you come?* His answer devastated me. *I am there, in you.* In frustration I cried out, *But what am I supposed to do?*

My search continued. Two things were clear in my mind:

1. Jesus healed sick persons two thousand years ago, usually working through their faith or through the faith of family or friends.

2. Medical science is now healing many persons who are sick, but not all, and in many cases it is healing them incompletely.

A serious question plagued me. Jesus not only healed sick persons himself; he also told his disciples to do the same, and they did. I was his disciple, and I was healing some of those who came to me. I was using medical science, which, of course, Jesus did not have available to him. However, where did faith come into the picture? Has medical technology supplanted faith? Or can medicine and faith come together and care for the whole person?

Medicine and the Person in Africa

A few years later I went with my family to Central Africa. Being the only physician in an active bush hospital, I had no time for language classes. I simply learned the Kituba language as I worked, primarily in the clinic. I quickly determined how to diagnose stomach trouble (gastritis): when someone, usually a woman, pointed to her lower chest and then patted her back between the shoulders, I knew immediately what the problem was. With limited language skills I became adept at prescribing sodium bicarbonate and belladonna extract, and then giving instructions to eat slowly, avoid hot spices, and have three meals a day (impossible for an African woman). It took years for me to learn that behind almost every case of "gastritis" was chronic anger, worry, fear, a broken relationship, or serious grief. A half a ton of sodium bicarbonate could never heal the real problems causing gastritis, for they lay beyond the scope of our biomedical model.

I remember patiently explaining to a seriously malnourished woman the kind of foods she needed to eat regularly to rebuild her body. When she returned to the clinic three weeks later with a joyful smile and looking vastly improved, I was surprised, for seldom did we see such rapid improvement with chronically malnourished persons. She explained that one of the nurses had introduced her to Jesus Christ, that Christ had come into her heart, and she had found real joy and peace. Her appetite had greatly improved, and she was feeling much stronger. As she left, I wondered what the relationship was between her new-found spiritual life and her nutritional status. It took me a long time to find out.

These cases are only a few among thousands that made me feel inadequate as a physician. Sitting in the clinic day after day, year after year, seeing so many persons with chronic complaints return time after time to receive the same medicines and instructions but experience no improvements whatsoever made me seriously question what I was accomplishing. The hospital was supposed to heal people, but it seemed more like a body and fender shop. I was supposed to be a physician, to be a healer, but I felt more like Mr. Fix-it, who often failed to fix the problem. I did not realize that the real problem needing to be fixed was in me. Yet the problem was not only in me; it was in the whole system of modern medical care.

The Spiritual Factor Emerging

Although I was a Christian practicing medicine, I did not know how faith fit into the practice of healing. I gave lip service to the truism that "we treat and God heals," but I had no idea how this worked. In 1984 a gifted young African woman—a pastor—joined our hospital staff. Mrs. Felicity Matala had just graduated from the Evangelical School of Theology in Kinshasa, where she had taken courses in hospital pastoral counseling. Mrs. Matala has an intimate personal relationship with Christ, a deep knowledge of the Bible, training in pastoral counseling, and gifts of listening, encouragement, and discernment. We (the staff physicians) and often our nurses began referring sick persons to her for counseling. Many had illnesses in which stress played an important role. Others had predominantly physical illnesses such as tuberculosis, cirrhosis, other chronic infections, even HIV/AIDS. We were impressed by the beneficial effects that occurred when sick persons went through the counseling process and found healing for emotions, feelings, and conflicts in relationships. We saw that their physical illnesses would often improve or heal more quickly.

We likewise discovered that spiritual rebirth—entering into a personal relationship with Jesus Christ—produced positive physical effects. We saw how prayer intervened in ways science could not explain. Were we seeing Christ heal as he once had healed in Galilee? We believed that this was so and that finally we were beginning to care for the whole person.

We also recognized the immense advantage of being able to work together as a healing team. We physicians had neither the time nor the training to help sick persons with their personal lives, their feelings, their emotions, and their relationships. Nor were we adequately equipped to enter into the time-consuming process of spiritual care.

Mrs. Matala and I realized that all of the hospital staff were involved in the caring process. Nurses spent far more time in personal contact with sick persons than physicians did (this is always the case, in any hospital or clinic). The operating room staff and the midwifery personnel were with sick persons at critical moments in their lives. They needed to know how to be effective helpers in caring for the whole person.

Beyond those people were personnel in other technical services, and even in the administration department. How they related to those who were ill could be of great importance to the outcome. If the very first contact person greeted a sick person warmly and with affirmation, this began building the level of confidence so necessary for effective caring.

So Mrs. Matala and I took time from our busy schedules to train many of the hospital personnel. The director of nursing, who had remarkable personal skills, assisted us. The training included student nurses, for they needed to learn these skills at the beginning of their professional careers. After a little while, as I walked through the wards, I would often see one of the staff or students talking quietly with a sick person or praying together. We realized that Mrs. Matala and her counseling team and the whole hospital staff were healers, and that care for the whole person was coming into place. Let me illustrate this with a case study.

Tuberculosis That Would Not Go Away

John came to our hospital a few years ago seriously ill with tuberculosis. Eighteen years old and a high school student, he had been ill for six months before coming to us. Although he was very sick, we were confident we could cure his disease. After all, we now have excellent medicines to treat tuberculosis. We hospitalized John and put him on the standard course of three antibiotics.

After one month of treatment, it was clear that John was not improving; instead, he was getting

sicker. We assumed it was because his tuberculosis bacilli were resistant to the antibiotics, so we switched
his treatment to more powerful and expensive ones.
These also had no effect. It soon became evident that
John was dying and we did not know the reason.

One day a nursing student discovered why John was
ill. She came to us and told us that John had been
cursed. John had wanted to attend high school, but
his parents had no money to pay the high school fees.
They had borrowed money from an uncle so that
John could go to high school. Some months later, the
uncle demanded reimbursement, but the poverty-
stricken parents did not have the money to pay him
back. The uncle became angry, and in the presence of
John he put a curse on him. He told the parents that
John had used up all his money. He would become ill
and, in spite of all the doctors might do for him, he
would die. That was exactly what John was doing before our very eyes in spite of the best available medical care.

For such a problem, physicians have no remedy. No
pills can cure a curse nor can a scalpel remove it. In
the African context, the curse is direct and is usually
taken literally. When that occurs, the result can be
devastating. In North American and European con-
texts, the curse is more indirect but can be just as
devastating. The words "cancer" or "AIDS" can act
like a curse. Even more so can statements like,
"You're no good. You will never succeed!" or "You
have an incurable disease," or "Get your affairs in order. You have only three months to live."

Mrs. Matala and our student nurse knew the solutions to John's problems. They introduced John to Jesus Christ, and within a short time John became a
Christian. We rejoiced, knowing that his eternal commitment to Christ reflected Christ's eternal commit-

ment to him. We had fulfilled our role as a traditional evangelical medical community. We had provided John the best medical care available and had led him to Jesus, the Great Physician. However, John was still dying of tuberculosis, a curable disease, and we did not know why. Mrs. Matala did, and she was not going to give up until John was fully healed.

She discerned that John had problems deeper than his tuberculosis, problems that his religious conversion had not resolved. She read to him of the power of Christ, how he healed the sick, calmed the storm, multiplied bread and fish, and even raised the dead. Then she asked John a simple question: "John, who is stronger, Jesus or your uncle?"

John immediately recognized that Jesus was stronger than his uncle. Mrs. Matala assured him that now he belonged to Christ and that the protective power of Christ in his heart was greater than the destructive power of his uncle to kill him. What she was doing was treating John's deep fear of the power of sorcery, and that fear was healed.

Mrs. Matala knew there was still more to be done. She asked John if he thought his uncle had done him wrong. John replied, "Of course he did me wrong. He tried to kill me." Mrs. Matala then explained how Christ commands us to forgive those who have wronged us. This was a much more difficult step for John to take, for how can we forgive those who intentionally wrong us and seem happy about it? Nevertheless, with the help of Mrs. Matala and others on the staff John was able, in prayer, to forgive his uncle. The anger and hatred in John's heart were thus healed. His fever soon disappeared, his appetite returned, he began to gain weight, and within a few months he had fully recovered. The spiritual factor, sound psychology, and good medical care had come together. John was healed in spirit, mind, and body, and he was restored to wholeness.

Disease and Illness

What happened here? Did John have a disease or was he ill? Was he cured, or was he healed? What is the difference between disease and illness, between being cured and being healed? Let's look at these questions to know what we are talking about.

A **disease** is *a particular condition* that upsets the well-functioning equilibrium of a person. Some diseases come into a person from the outside—an infection, an accident, or an intoxication by a harmful substance. Other diseases are the result of changes within the person. Something has upset the body's normal, healthy equilibrium. High blood pressure and diabetes are examples of this kind of disease. Malignant tumors come from changes in cell function whereby certain cells begin growing in chaotic fashion.

We know a lot about diseases that come in from the outside. We know much less about diseases that come from changes in our organs, mechanisms, or cells. Why do small arteries become constricted and cause high blood pressure? Why does the pancreas no longer produce enough insulin? Why do normal cells become abnormal and develop into cancer?

Illness on the other hand *has to do with the person*. Illness is all the uncomfortable, disturbing things that happen to and within a person when a disease is present. John had tuberculosis, a disease. However, John himself was ill, and his illness was much more than just the action of the tuberculosis bacilli on the tissues and organs of his body. It affected his whole being, including his thoughts, feelings, emotions, and spirit, the very center of his personality.

Curing and Healing

Curing has to do with disease. **Healing** has to do with illness. While curing means getting rid of the disease, healing restores the person to health. Some diseases we can cure. We can cure tuberculosis and many other infections, and sometimes even cancer. Other diseases, such as HIV/AIDS and many cancers, we cannot cure. Yet even in these incurable situations, we can help a person become less ill by healing the thoughts, feelings, emotions, relationships, and spirit. The disease may still be present and even increasing, yet the mind and spirit of the sick person can be healed and restored to productive, creative functioning. What is exciting to see is that when the healing of heart, mind, and spirit occur, even so-called incurable diseases may diminish and sometimes even disappear.

Problems in Caregiving

We want to bring together the curing of disease and the healing of persons. We want to care for the whole person: body, mind, and spirit. But there are big obstacles to this. First of all, caregiving in this age—and particularly in Western cultures—has become very compartmentalized. One kind of caregiver tends to the body (and specialists care for specific parts of the body and specific systems in the body); another kind of caregiver focuses on the mental and emotional state of a person; yet another kind of caregiver, usually a pastor, tends to the spiritual aspects of a person. Most of the time, these different caregivers never meet one another, let alone consult about the one person all three of them may be treating at the same time.

Medical doctors, nurses, technicians, physical therapists, psychologists, psychiatrists, therapists, social workers, counselors, pastors, and the many others who might care for a person—all receive training within their own fields. They have their own offices or clinics in which they do their healing work. But the overall system is not set up for these caregivers to work together, even though the people they try to help often need help from all of them. If I (the physician) feel you need to see a psychologist or a pastoral counselor, this requires a second appointment and probably a second trip somewhere, perhaps across town. It likewise involves additional fees. So besides the geographical separation of caregivers, we add an economic obstacle as well. And even if I do refer you to a psychologist or a pastoral counselor, I usually will not follow up on that consultation, nor will I hear back from him or her. I am caring for part of you, and someone else is caring for another part of you.

Yet, healing of the whole person requires a concerted, coordinated effort by each of the many people who are trained, gifted—and yes, called—to be healers.

The Spiritual Factor: Faith

The second great obstacle to comprehensive healing of the person is the neglect of spiritual resources. All of us caregivers are using sophisticated technology and, particularly in psychology and therapy, complex philosophical models. Yet we limit ourselves to technologies and models.

The essential ingredient that is missing is faith, that intangible ingredient of the heart that includes trust and commitment. Faith is a relationship, and the ultimate relationship is to a Power beyond ourselves, to God, who can help us bring all things together. I am writing as a Christian, and I am writing about how faith—trust in and commitment to Jesus Christ—can bring wholeness to mind and spirit and through that can promote healing of the body.

The power of Jesus to heal is a real power, and it is outside the human psyche. The words of Jesus can help us psychologically, and so can the words of the Bible. Even more, the presence of the spirit of Jesus Christ within us can bring healing to the spirit. When Jesus enters the personality by our invitation (and that is the only way he can enter), he can then make available to us his power to heal the heart, mind, soul, and spirit, and through that give strength to the body.

For me the spiritual factor is bringing Jesus Christ into the healing process. It is making Christ's power available to all who understand and want it so that Christ can work alongside the powers of medicine and psychology to care for the whole person. This spiritual dimension is what I see missing in medicine and even in many Christian ministries of healing, including my own for many years.

We diverse caregivers need to come together and work as a team. If we then bring faith in Christ into our practices, we will be bringing together what is necessary to care for the whole person: body, mind, and spirit. That is what this book is about.

John's real problem was a social problem, a conflict between his parents and his uncle. The uncle's curse became a spiritual illness for John. John believed he would become ill and would die, so the meaning and purpose of his life were destroyed. Mrs. Matala and some of the nurses brought Jesus into John's life, and the presence of Christ in his heart healed his spirit and gave him new meaning and purpose for life. Then the words of Jesus as recorded in the Bible healed him psychologically by enabling him to overcome his fear and anger and to forgive his uncle. Now John's body was able to respond, and he got well. John himself was healed. This included being cured of his tuberculosis, a cure that we physicians with our medical skills and resources could not make happen by ourselves.

John's story shows how medicine, counseling, and faith in Jesus Christ can work together, in one place, to restore a person to wholeness. Can we explain this scientifically as well as biblically? Let's look first at how Jesus himself healed sick persons.

2

Words That Heal

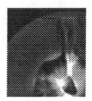

The Gospel writers clearly show that when Jesus healed a person who was ill, he intended to heal the whole person. He wanted to restore body, mind, and spirit, and make it possible for the person to return to his or her family and community.

A Woman with a "Gynecological Problem"

How did Jesus heal the whole person? And how can Jesus heal each of us, whatever our situation? We find the following story in Mark's Gospel, chapter 5.

> There was a woman who had suffered terribly from severe bleeding for twelve years, even though she had been treated by many doctors. She had spent all her money, but instead of getting better she got worse all the time. She had heard about Jesus, so she came in the crowd behind him, saying to herself, "If I just touch his clothes, I will get well."

> She touched his cloak, and the bleeding stopped at once; and she had the feeling inside herself that she was healed of her trouble. At once Jesus knew that power had gone out of him, so he turned in the crowd and asked, "Who touched my clothes?" His disciples answered, "You see how people are crowding you; why do you ask who touched you?"

> But Jesus kept looking around to see who had done it. The woman realized what had happened to her, so she came, trembling with fear, knelt at his feet, and told him the whole truth. Jesus said to her, "My daughter, your faith has made you well. Go in peace, and be healed of your trouble." (vv. 25-34)

Before examining this story, let's look at three principles of Bible interpretation. First of all, although the Bible is composed of many books, those books are a unified whole. Many Old Testament concepts illuminate or illustrate New Testament truths. An Old Testament passage will shed important light on this story.

Second, we must know the cultural context of the passage. What were the beliefs, attitudes, and practices of the people among whom the story took place or to whom the passage was written? How did they understand the story or the message? Jesus was a Jew. This woman was a Jew, and Jewish culture played a strong role in this drama.

Third, God has given us common sense and imagination, and he expects us to use both as we approach the Scriptures. Many stories contain few details, only the bare essentials. By using reason, imagination, and the leading of the Holy Spirit, we can add other details to the story which, although not included in the written text, were most likely present. In other words, with inspired imagination, we can read between the lines.

The Physical Context

This woman had suffered from irregular bleeding for twelve years. Mark gives no indication of the cause. It surely was not a malignant tumor, because cancer progresses to death much more rapidly. Furthermore, cancer of the uterus is rare among Jewish women. It is likely that the bleeding was due to a long-standing imbalance in her hormones. Pain probably accompanied the bleeding, making her life miserable. She was most certainly anemic because of this chronic blood loss. As such, she was weak and could not carry on the daily work of the home and family. I assume she had no children during those twelve difficult years because, with the irregularity of her menstrual cycle, she could not conceive. Infertility was a very serious problem for Jewish women, as it is for most women in any culture.

Here then is the physical context: a woman with a serious gynecological problem.

The Social Context

This Jewish woman was subject to Jewish culture and the Old Testament Law. According to the Levitical law, which we find in Leviticus 15:19-30, a woman was unclean during her normal menstrual period and for seven days thereafter. She was also unclean any time irregular bleeding occurred. Furthermore, she made unclean all her clothes, her house, any furniture or objects she touched, and anyone with whom she came in contact. So for twelve years this woman had been unclean and had rendered the world around her unclean. If she had been married, her husband certainly had divorced her. Her family had abandoned her, and she had no friends. How could she have friends if they were constantly in danger of becoming unclean? Finally, Mark says she was penniless, having spent all her money on futile attempts to be cured.

The Spiritual Context

Probably this woman's heaviest burden was her spiritual situation. Because she was unclean, she could not go to the temple to worship God. She could not go to pray, to give an offering, or even to plead for help. Socially she was all alone and without resources; spiritually she was cut off from God and was in despair. So Mark is not describing for us simply a "gynecological problem." Mark speaks truly when he says, "There was a *woman* who had suffered terribly." She had suffered in the totality of her life.

One day this woman heard about Jesus, a powerful man who could heal the sick. Hope dawned in her heart. However, she could not go to Jesus to ask for help. No Jewish woman could go to a strange man either to converse with him or to ask for anything. If she did, she would be considered immoral. Furthermore, in her condition she would render this important man unclean. Another man—her husband, a brother, a friend—could go to Jesus and intercede for her. But this woman was completely abandoned and had no one to help her or to find help for her. Yet she was not ready to give up. She determined to cast herself at the mercy of this man Jesus, whoever he might be.

She came up with a plan that was both desperate and dangerous. She would come up behind Jesus, in the middle of a crowd of people, and touch his clothes. Secrecy was absolutely essential for her, because if anyone observed her, she would be publicly accused of defiling Jesus and perhaps even stoned to death. But in many ways she was already dead, so what did she have to lose?

When she touched Jesus' cloak, she immediately felt something in her body. It might have been a sudden feeling of warmth, or the sensation of an organ contracting. Whatever it was, it was a perceptible physical change in her body. What joy she must have felt for an instant, because she knew she was healed! Now she must escape immediately. But that was impossible. This man Jesus exposed her. She had insulted him. She had made him unclean. Furthermore, she had stolen his power and somehow he knew it. Now he was calling her, and she would probably be stoned. So, as Mark described, she came terror-stricken, fell at Jesus' feet, and told him the whole story.

Why did Jesus expose this woman? He knew that someone had been physically healed, for as Mark says, he "knew that power had gone out of him." We physicians are usually delighted when we have healed someone. Could Jesus not be content with that? No, because the *woman herself* had not been healed. Jesus had healed her female organs but had not yet healed her as a person, and so he called her to him. As she lay prostrate on the ground before Jesus, awaiting the word of her condemnation, she heard an absolutely incredible Aramaic word which is translated, "My daughter." "My daughter" she heard Jesus say to her gently, and that word healed her.

For thirty-five years I practiced medicine and surgery in Africa. I cared for countless numbers of women with bleeding problems and infertility. I performed hundreds, perhaps thousands, of operations on them. But how often did I speak a word that healed the whole person, that restored to health the spirit, mind, and emotions of the one who was ill?

The Healing Word

What heals the broken heart and the wounded spirit? What is the "intervention" necessary for this? We have many inventories for healing the body, but what heals the heart?

What heals the heart is simply a word spoken to the depths of the sick person's spirit. It is that key word or phrase that the person's spirit understands in such a way as to resolve all the psycho-spiritual problems—the fear, conflicts, anxiety, guilt, and despair. When this word heals the inner pain, the whole inner self is restored.

Even after her internal organs had been healed, this woman was still ill psychologically, socially, and spiritually, because all her relationships remained broken. What Jesus said to this woman spoke to the depths of her heart and healed those broken relationships. With her ears she heard Jesus say, "My daughter." In her spirit she heard him say, "I love you. I accept you. You are worthy to live in my family. You are now healed and made whole." This word restored her relationship with herself. She knew that somehow, in the eyes of this marvelous man named Jesus, she was worthy. Her dignity was restored, and immediately the fear, rejection, and despair that had destroyed her life were removed.

This word likewise opened for her a brand-new spiritual relationship. She entered into a relationship with her Maker through the person of Jesus Christ. Now she belonged to the family of God, the family to which she (and all of us) should have belonged from the time of conception. Now she could pray, worship, offer her gifts, and lay her sins and imperfections at his feet. Life had new meaning for her.

When Jesus said to her, "Go in peace, and be healed of your trouble," her social relationships were also healed. This meant she was clean and could now live with others. All of her disgrace was gone and she could rejoin her family, her friends, and her community. Social healing is as important as any other aspect of our restoration, and Jesus accomplished that with this woman.

Human life *is* relationships. The Christian life is right relationships. True healing restores hurting or broken relationships, and Jesus restored those relationships in the life of this woman.

A Woman with a Broken Heart

Let me bring this principle back to our present world by telling you about another Jewish woman with a similar story. Deborah is a dynamic and attractive Jewish lawyer. But she almost died of a broken heart.

Deborah grew up in a nonreligious Jewish family, although as a girl she enjoyed reading the Psalms and the Prophets. After law school she married a Gentile lawyer and they had two children. Unfortunately the marriage soon went from tumultuous to acrimonious and was terminated when her husband abandoned her for a pretty secretary. Imagine the trauma: a lovely, intelligent, capable Jewish woman despised and rejected by the man to whom she had made a lifelong commitment. Her heart was filled with shame, anger, grief, loneliness, and a deep sense of the "one flesh" marriage union being torn apart. As a single parent, she could not keep up with a demanding law practice, and she had no way to support herself and her children. Her life shattered, she began contemplating suicide.

In her misery she went to visit a friend, who gave her a Bible and suggested she read about Jesus. With her Jewish background and knowledge of the culture, Deborah saw in the Gospel accounts many things Gentiles do not see. When she read the story of this woman with bleeding, she totally identified with her. Deborah's heart was bleeding, and her life also had been destroyed. Then she read what this woman did and she was shocked. No Jewish woman could ever do that! The man Jesus, being Jewish, would have to destroy her; the religious code demanded it.

When Deborah read what Jesus said to the woman, that instead of condemning her he called her "My daughter," she was overwhelmed. She said to herself, *If Jesus could call that woman "My daughter," he could call me his daughter too.* She fell on her knees and prayed, "Jesus, I don't know who you are, but I want to be your daughter." In the depths of her heart she heard him say, "Deborah, you are my daughter." In that moment, Deborah was healed by the same word Jesus had spoken to another woman two thousand years ago.

From the Mind to the Heart

What is this word that can heal the broken heart or the wounded spirit? It can be a single word, such as the Aramaic word, "My daughter." It may be a longer explanation, or instructions, or a story. It can be a passage from the Bible, a word spoken in prayer, or a message spoken to the heart by the Holy Spirit. It can also be a visible image or a symbol that, when perceived by the deep mind, resolves inner conflicts and brings peace and healing.

God, knowing the stubbornness of the hearts of the children of Israel, explained this principle to the prophet Isaiah in a negative way:

> God said, "Go and tell this people: 'You will be ever hearing, but never understanding; you will be ever seeing, but never perceiving.' This people's heart has become calloused; they hardly hear with their ears, and they have closed their eyes. Otherwise, they might see with their eyes, hear with their ears, understand with their hearts, and turn and be healed." (Isaiah 6:9-10, Septuagint translation)

The message of the text is clear. What we hear and see goes into our mind. If these thoughts are understood and accepted by our feelings, emotions, and intuition, healing can occur. It is significant that this passage is quoted by all four of the Gospel writers and by the apostle Paul.[1]

While our intellect deals primarily with ideas, our heart is more often moved by symbols. Symbols help us understand reality at deeper levels than mere words can address. When information changes from a mere idea to a symbol, then our feelings, emotions, and intuition can understand it. The woman with bleeding heard Jesus call her his daughter. This idea did not correspond to reality, because Jesus was not her biological father. Her heart, however, immediately understood the symbolism as she perceived Jesus receiving her into his family, affirming her, and making her pure. In the same way, Deborah, overwhelmed by Jesus' acceptance of this woman, reached out desperately to him and asked him to call her his daughter. When her heart perceived him accepting her as his daughter, she also was healed and her life was transformed.

The Power of Words

Words have power. They can heal, build up, and strengthen us. Or they can inflict pain, provoke illness, and even destroy life. Chapter 1 tells about John, who suffered from tuberculosis. He had heard a destroying word from his uncle—"You will die"—and John almost did die. However, John committed his life to Christ and was then able to hear healing words that were more powerful than the destructive words of his uncle.

Mrs. Matala asked John a question: "Who is stronger, Jesus or your uncle?" John's intellect processed that question on the basis of what he had heard from Mrs. Matala and what he had read in the Bible. When he replied, "Jesus is stronger," he spoke a healing word to his own heart, which understood that he now had no further reason to fear his uncle. Mrs. Matala then helped John recognize his need to forgive his uncle. In prayer, he told God he had forgiven his uncle. John's heart understood that word and let go of the anger and hatred to which he was clinging. His heart was thus healed and began to strengthen his body. We will see in chapter 4 how this process works.

Norman Cousins has written a significant book entitled *The Healing Heart*. In the introduction, Dr. Bernard Lown, then professor of cardiology in Harvard University School of Medicine, recounts the story of a critically ill man who had just suffered a massive heart attack. In spite of intensive therapy, he seemed to be approaching his final moments. As Dr. Lown was listening to the man's heart, he detected an ominous rhythm in the heartbeat, a triple beat called a "gallop." Believing the man to be in coma, Dr. Lown called to his residents to come and listen to what he called "a wholesome gallop rhythm." Slowly and unexpectedly, the man improved and eventually recovered from his heart attack.

Some months later, when the man returned for a check-up, Dr. Lown remarked about his miraculous recovery. The man said, "Doctor, I not only know what got me better, but even the exact moment it happened. I was sure the end was near and that you and your staff had given up hope. However, Thursday morning, when you entered with your troops, something happened that changed everything. You listened to my heart; you seemed pleased by the findings and announced to all those standing about my bed that I had a 'wholesome gallop'. I knew that the doctors, in talking to me, might try to soften things. But they wouldn't kid each other. So when I overheard you tell your colleagues I had a wholesome gallop, I figured I still had a lot of kick to my heart and could not be dying. My spirits for the first time were lifted, and I knew I would live and recover."[2]

Words have the potential to damage life as well. Dr. Lown writes about a woman, Mrs. S, who had lived for years with a mild form of tricuspid stenosis (T.S.), a constricted valve in the heart. One day the then-professor of cardiology, who had followed Mrs. S's condition for years and knew her well, remarked in her presence to a large group of visiting physicians that she had T.S. He then left the room.

Within minutes Mrs. S's whole demeanor changed. She rapidly went into heart failure and died within twenty-four hours. Before she died, she whispered to Dr. Lown that, to her, T.S. meant "terminal situation." In spite of all possible reassurances, her spirit interpreted the word of the cardiologist to mean she was dying, and her physical heart responded by going into failure.[3]

God speaks to us in symbols. He has given us a multitude of symbols that can encourage and heal us. We can find these in his acts in history, in what the prophets, poets, and apostles have declared, and in what Christ has accomplished for our healing—in Gethsemane, on the cross, and by rising from the dead. We will be exploring these symbols in greater detail in chapter 6. More symbols come to us from the Holy Spirit, who is like a stream of water flowing through the hearts of all who are open to him.

A Healing Team

Why do health professionals today have such difficulty in caring for the whole person? Why do so few of us know how to speak words of healing to the hearts of people who are ill, or to find the symbols for which their hearts are searching? I am convinced that many Christian health professionals are willing, even anxious, to do this, but they do not know how. Our rationalistic and compartmentalized view of the world has made this integrated approach to healing very difficult. Furthermore, few physicians have the time to uncover the deep personal problems of those who consult us, or to discern the word or symbols necessary to heal these inner problems.

When Mrs. Matala came onto the staff of our hospital, she had both the training and the skills to discern inner situations and find the healing symbols for them. Furthermore, she had the time, and such work requires much time and patience. As physicians refer sick persons to her, she asks them questions and listens to their personal problems. She tries to discern the real problems of their minds and spirits. In talking with sick persons, she frequently uses a marvelous verse from the Bible, Proverbs 14:30: "Peace of mind makes the body healthy, but jealousy is like a cancer." She explains that cancer destroys the body. The Bible says that jealousy does the same thing. Not only jealousy, but envy, bitterness, fear, guilt, chronic anger, and all other destructive emotions. We call her our "heart doctor."

Often Mrs. Matala will gently introduce a sick person to the Lord Jesus Christ, and many of them are drawn into a relationship with him. Then she shows them how to unload their hurts, their pain, and their brokenness on Jesus and find the healing, peace, and restoration he can bring. Often physical illnesses are resolved in the process, and the whole person is healed. Even persons with AIDS find hope, renewed strength, and new life by coming to Jesus. As far as we know, none of them have been cured of the AIDS virus, but many of those with HIV do go into remission. Some live for months and others for years only by the power of God working through a heart that has been healed and is at peace.

We return now to the question of how Jesus healed—and if he can heal people today. We tend to think that all of Jesus' healings were miracles. By this we mean events that are unpredictable, that cannot be explained by known scientific laws, and that are therefore an intervention by God's power. We cannot replicate miracles. Jesus did perform many miracles, including miracles of healing, and we cannot explain them by physical or psychological laws that we know. For example, it is difficult to squeeze into a scientific framework the healing of a withered hand (Luke 6:6-11). Nor can we explain scientifically how the Roman centurion's servant suddenly recovered from his illness at the very moment that Jesus, some distance away, pronounced him healed (Matthew 8:5-13).

Yet it is a mistake to consider all of Jesus' healing works only as miracles and therefore beyond our capacity to replicate. I cannot explain scientifically how Jesus healed the gynecological problem of the woman with bleeding. However, I believe he brought together spiritual, psychological, and social dynamics with such power that he was able to heal her wholly. I believe these same dynamics are available to us today, and that Jesus' healing power can work through us.

A Man with Liver Disease

A man whom we will call Roger came to our hospital in the Congo last year. For two years he had suffered from vague abdominal pain, weakness, poor appetite, and weight loss. When I examined him, I found that he had an enlarged, hard, knobby, somewhat tender liver. We see much cirrhosis and liver cancer in Central Africa due to hepatitis B, and I assumed he had one or the other of these incurable and usually fatal conditions. As a physician I had little to offer him, but I did prescribe aspirin and some multivitamins. We have to give sick persons something to take; if not, they will be dissatisfied. I then suggested to him that he go to Mrs. Matala. I gave him a sealed note explaining to Mrs. Matala that Roger's prognosis was poor and that he needed counsel in preparation for dying.

A week later Roger returned to see me, stating that he felt much better. I thought, *Wonderful. Those vitamins really must have helped him!* When I examined his abdomen, to my astonishment, his hard, knobby, tender liver now appeared to be normal. I rechecked his chart, for I could hardly believe he was the same man

I had seen the week before. The name was correct, the address was correct, and I had actually drawn a picture of his big liver. This was indeed Roger. At that moment Mrs. Matala opened the door to tell me something. I invited her in and asked, "What in the world did you do for this man's liver?" She smiled and told me to come by her office when I had completed my rounds at the clinic.

Later, she told me about Roger. She had spent hours with him as he described the shambles of his life: alcohol, drugs, promiscuous sexual behavior, witchcraft, and even open conflict with the chief of his village—very dangerous behavior in that culture. He was living in mortal fear of witchcraft and had a heavy burden of guilt. As Proverbs 14:30 tells us, destructive emotions destroy the body; Roger's liver had indeed begun the process of self-destruction.

After Roger had spilled out the problems in his life, Mrs. Matala talked to him about Jesus Christ and his power to heal the spirit. Roger committed his life to Christ and discovered a peace he had never known before. Then Mrs. Matala led him through the problems he had recounted, one by one. Roger confessed his sins of sexual infidelity and promiscuity, and Mrs. Matala gave him the healing word of assurance that his sins were forgiven. He forgave others who had wronged him, and healing came to his anger and hatred. His fear was resolved when Mrs. Matala explained that the power of the Holy Spirit in his heart was greater than the powers of witchcraft, sorcery, and magic. They discussed his problems of alcohol and drugs. When he asked Christ for help in overcoming them, Mrs. Matala prayed for his deliverance from their power. The words of that prayer penetrated Roger's heart and brought a feeling of freedom. In ways that we will discuss later, changes then occurred in the physical functioning of Roger's organs. Among other changes, his adrenal glands stopped over-producing hormones that cause inflammation. The inflammation of his liver disappeared, and it once again became normal. Roger was made whole.

This is a story of God's power working through the spirit and mind of a sick man *to produce physical changes in his body.* The dynamics are similar to those Jesus used two thousand years ago. Words of healing spoken by Mrs. Matala were an important part of that process.

It is likewise a vivid story of how our lifestyle affects our health. Lifestyle problems can even produce physical disease of the body, as they did in this man. Furthermore, dealing with lifestyle problems openly, realistically, and with the help of God can be a crucial part of healing, even the physical healing of diseases.

The Bible clearly describes examples of Jesus healing diseases such as leprosy, blindness, and paralysis. The story of Roger and the healing of his liver, and also of John and his recovery from tuberculosis, are examples of such healing occurring today. Most certainly this does not occur in all cases; in fact, it is still unusual. Yet the healing of the inner life does two things:

1. It releases the body from the negative influences that painful or destructive emotions can produce.

2. It adds positive influences that can reinforce the recuperative powers of the body.

So even though physical healing does not always occur, or does not occur immediately, *the healing of the heart, mind, and spirit creates a favorable environment in which the body can respond to the challenges of the disease process.* In some cases (though by no means all), this bodily response can result in physical healing. We will now look at how this takes place.

3

God Made Us Whole

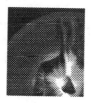

Amiddle-aged man, Aaron, came to our hospital complaining of pain that he had had for six years in the lower abdomen. The only antecedent I could get from his history was that he had had a brief episode of gonorrhea at the beginning of his illness. Although he had received good antibiotic treatment for this, and all signs of infection had disappeared, his pain persisted. He had been to many hospitals and clinics and had received many different antibiotics, all to no avail. Various possibilities ran through my mind: a focus of resistant infection, a tumor, or a bone or joint problem. However, I could find no physical signs of disease to explain his pain. All of his laboratory examinations were normal, including a test for HIV. I referred him to Mrs. Matala, our pastoral counselor.

Mrs. Matala took a history from Aaron, as I had done. She then began asking him about his work, his living conditions, and his feelings about this illness. When she asked him about his marriage, he burst into tears and said, "Mrs. Matala, I know why I hurt." With considerable difficulty he told her that he had betrayed his wife six years previously while on a trip, and ever since that time he'd had pain. He said that he was not an immoral man; this was the only time he had fallen to temptation. Yet he knew he had done wrong, and now he realized that this was why he was hurting.

After listening, without comment, to Aaron's story, Mrs. Matala began asking questions about his spiritual life. Had he found any help from his faith in God? She determined that he had no real faith in Jesus Christ, and so she described what it means to have a personal relationship with Christ. She explained how Christ died for our sins so that he could truly forgive us the wrongs we do and then take away our hurt, pain, and guilt. Aaron asked Christ to come into his heart, and Mrs. Matala helped him confess his sins to Jesus. Using 1 John 1:9 as her authority, she assured Aaron that his sins were forgiven, including his sin against his wife. This word of forgiveness was the word Aaron's heart needed, and almost immediately his lower abdominal pain disappeared.

This is a rather strange story, isn't it? Aaron had real pain in his lower abdomen. When I pressed on that area, he hurt. Yet there was no physical cause for this pain—no infection or abscess. Was it all "in his head"? No, it was in his heart. Now, how in the world can a "heart problem" cause pain in the abdomen? This chapter and the next will focus on that question.

What was the physical cause of Aaron's pain? It might have been muscle tension or spasms in the area associated with his old infection. Or it could have been a non-infectious inflammatory process in that area. Whatever it was, the real cause was a feeling of guilt that reminded him of his old infection and the wrongdoing that had caused it. When his heart accepted the forgiveness of Christ and stopped accusing him, the tension, spasms, inflammation, or whatever was wrong went away.

Created by God

In the book of Genesis we read that God took natural physical elements, such as soil, and with them made this amazingly complex body of ours. The Bible gives no details, but anyone who has ever studied the human body cannot help but be deeply moved by its marvelous intricacy. I have often wondered how many "God-hours" the Almighty used to put together our arteries, veins, and capillaries; our muscles, tendons, and ligaments; our bones, joints, and nerves; our brain, spinal cord, and organs of sense. Furthermore, the astoundingly complex relationships between all our organ systems stretch our analytical capacities to the limit.

Nevertheless, when God had completed this amazing masterpiece, it had no life. Something was missing, namely the breath of life, and so God breathed his spirit into this first physical being. The body then became a living being, a person (Genesis 2:7).

In medical school almost fifty years ago, the professor of biochemistry announced to us one day that within a few years we would be able to explain all of human activity by means of enzymes. My spirit shuddered. I knew I was much more than a collection of biochemical enzymes, and to this day I have never found out how many enzymes it requires to make a human spirit or to generate a thought or a feeling! The Bible makes it clear that without the breath of life, without spirit, we are not living beings. Something in the depths of our heart resonates with that, and that "something" is what we call spirit. It was not Aaron's enzymes that were reacting to his sinful act; it was his spirit. His heart was transferring his spiritual pain to his lower abdomen in ways we will describe later.

Body, Soul, and Spirit

Elsewhere the Bible speaks about body, soul, and spirit (1 Thessalonians 5:23). The Bible is not a dictionary. It does not "define" these terms; in fact, it often uses them interchangeably. Definitions are limiting, and the terms soul, mind, spirit, heart, and even body are far too dynamic to have parameters fixed around them. But for the purposes of this book, I'll explain what I mean by this terminology.

The body is the physical area of life. It has to do with protoplasm, proteins, carbohydrates, and fat, all put together in a host of complex cells. These cells are organized into tissues, organs, and groups of organs that enable us to function. The term "physiological" refers to the functioning of these physical elements. On some occasions, the Bible uses the word "body" to refer to the physical body. On other occasions "body" refers to the whole person. The Bible sometimes uses bones to refer to the whole body or even the whole person.

The mind is the intellectual area of life where we do our thinking, analyzing, and reflecting. We call this the conscious mind, and it is the domain of the intellect, reason, logic, analysis, synthesis, and judgment. Our perceptions of the world around us come into the mind, where they are transposed into impressions, thoughts, and ideas.

The affect is our feelings, emotions, attitudes, and intuitions. Our beliefs and desires are here as well as our memories. This is where the thoughts and ideas of the intellect are processed, understood, and assimilated or rejected. The affect involves the nervous system; it also influences and is influenced by the other organs and bodily systems. We often call this the subconscious mind.

I use the word soul to embrace both the mind and the affect. We also refer to the mind and the affect as the psyche. The term psychological refers to the functioning of the mind and the affect. We cannot separate mind and affect, any more than we can tease apart our thoughts, feelings, and emotions. They all go together to make up the soul.

The spirit is the center of the personality. It is in my spirit that I ask the basic questions of life: Who am I? Why am I here? Where am I going? It is in my spirit that I try to find meaning and purpose. My spirit seeks to determine where I am going and how I will get there. It is in my spirit that I make the key decisions of my life. By my spirit, I come into relationship with those invisible spiritual and personal powers that surround me—God and all that comes from him, or the spiritual powers of evil. Through my spirit I am in touch with powers that influence my life, and by my spirit I can influence others around me.

The Bible often combines the concepts of soul and spirit in one term, the heart. In this sense it is not the muscular organ responsible for the circulation of our blood. It signifies the center of our personality and includes the soul and spirit; in this sense, "heart" refers to our nonmaterial inner self.

Social relationships make up another major dimension of our life. We live in a web of relationships. We belong to a family of one sort or another. We relate to friends, neighbors, work associates, and strangers. We are part of our culture, and our frames of reference come largely from our culture and social relationships. When things go wrong in our relationships with others, this affects our health and can cause illness.

What we have described here is our inner life. It is the invisible and intangible aspect of us that is nevertheless absolutely real. It is our real self. Without this inner self our physical body is but a lump of clay. How do our invisible inner life and our visible physical body fit together?

The Bible says, "Above all else, guard your heart, for it is the wellspring of life" (Proverbs 4:23, NIV). That includes the health and strength of our body. How we guard and nourish the image of God in our inner life is of great importance to our health, and we turn to that now.

The Image of God and Our Health

God has created us in his image. This is an essential aspect of our humanity that is not studied in medical schools. It is discussed in theological schools, but seldom if ever do theologians consider how it relates to our health or healing.

Genesis 1:26-27 tells us that God made us "in his image." Volumes have been written about the imago dei, and we will not attempt to synthesize them here. However, knowing that we bear the image of God should indicate to us some fundamental aspects of our personality—and our healing.

Our nature as persons comes from God, bears his image, and is therefore good

This nature includes

- our creativity
- our social or relational nature, and our need and capacity to communicate with others
- our intellect, reason, and ability to figure things out

- our imagination
- our emotions and intuition
- our joy and appreciation of beauty
- our sexuality, for masculinity and femininity both come from God

God has made us like himself, not in degree but in quality

Although we are finite, we are of infinite worth no matter what our current condition may be.

Each of us needs healing because the image of God within us has been marred

The process of healing is therefore the process of restoring the image of God within us. Although that image will not be fully restored in this life, the goal of healing is to help us become more and more like our Maker.

Why is it important for us to understand what it means to be in the image of God? Let me suggest three reasons.

Jesus understood the image of God in persons

Even in someone whose body was terribly disfigured by leprosy, he saw a person who bore the image of God. Jesus saw God's image in a woman whose compulsive sexual behavior brought her to the point of being stoned to death by the religious leaders. Instead of condemning her, he affirmed her as a person and set her free (John 8:1-11).

No disease of the body or illness of the soul can destroy God's image within us

Cancer, HIV/AIDS, and a multitude of other destructive diseases can distort God's image, but never destroy it. In whatever physical, mental, or social situation we may be, we bear and always will bear the image of our Maker, and Jesus wants to restore it to its original perfection.

Our very awareness of God's image within us provides potent power for healing
To be like God is our destiny. Our goal should be to become more and more like him. This is an attainable hope because God has promised to work in us, if we want him to, to make us like himself.[1] Illness distorts God's image in us if it brings into the soul fear, anger, shame, bitterness, or depression. But knowing what I am to be like and that somehow this illness can be a means of helping me get there can restore my soul and help my body.

"Inasmuch . . ."

When I went into the emergency room of our hospital in the Congo one morning, I saw an unusual looking man lying on one of the beds. He was emaciated, disheveled, and dirty, and I had trouble seeing the image of God in him. The head nurse told me, "This is Mr. Abdul. He is Egyptian, and he is very sick." I sat by his bedside to find out about his illness and his life.

Mr. Abdul, a Muslim, told me he had fled Egypt fifteen years ago for political reasons. He had been in the Congo ever since and was involved in the diamond trade. In the past year he had become increasingly ill, and he was sure he had tuberculosis. After examining him, I requested a chest X-ray and blood serology for HIV infection. I asked Mrs. Matala to visit him. She spent an hour with him in a time of spiritual care and sharing, and he asked her to pray with him.

When I went to the radiology lab later to look at

Mr. Abdul's chest film, the technician smiled and said, "Do you know what we call this man? We call him Jesus." She explained that the staff thought Mr. Abdul's ruddy brown complexion, long wavy black hair, and beard resembled their concept of Jesus. "OK, please show me 'Jesus'' chest film," I said. The film showed that his lungs were clear. "Jesus" had no signs of tuberculosis.

I next went to the laboratory to find the results of his blood test for AIDS. The staff there said, "You mean the test of the man we call Jesus?" I opened the locked cabinet and looked at Mr. Abdul's blood sample number; the result was marked positive.

I found Mrs. Matala and informed her that Mr. Abdul had AIDS. Together we returned and sat by his bedside. Gently I told him the good news: he did not have tuberculosis. Then I gave him the bad news: he did have another more serious infection caused by the AIDS virus. The two of us explained to him the living hope available to all persons, even to those with HIV, the hope of real and eternal life in Jesus. Mr. Abdul's gratitude was amazing; he thanked us profusely for telling him the truth about his condition and also about Christ. Again he asked us to pray with him. He then asked if he could return to Kinshasa to be with his wife and children.

The following day I was to fly into Kinshasa on the Mission Aviation Fellowship plane, and one other seat was available. Mr. Abdul went with me, and when we landed in Kinshasa, his family was there to meet him. After he thanked me again, we said goodbye, and he disappeared into the crowd accompanied by his family. At that moment a familiar voice spoke quietly in the depths of my spirit. "Your nurses were right. In caring for this man, you cared for me. 'Inasmuch as you did this for one of the least important of these brothers of mine, you did it for me!'" (Matthew 26:40). The tears that fell on the tarmac were those of grief mingled with thanksgiving. I hope to see Mr. Abdul again. The image of God within him had indeed been marred by many circumstances, but the Lord was restoring that image.

The two most exciting adventures of life are these:

- to permit God to work in our life toward the restoration of his image in us
- to permit God to work through us to help restore his image in other people

To be healed means much more than to be cured of a disease. When we are healed, we are restored as people in whom God's image is being renewed. Even if the disease of the body remains, the renewal of God's image in heart, mind, soul, and spirit is always possible and should be our goal.

4

The Chemistry of Emotions

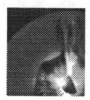

Medical science is becoming increasingly aware of how all aspects of our lives fit together. What happens in one area of life affects all other areas. A physical illness, like cancer or tuberculosis, stirs up many emotions—fear, frustration, even despair. On the other hand, fear or anger can upset digestion; anxiety can cause diarrhea; worry can generate headaches and even high blood pressure. When one part of the body suffers, the whole person is ill. How does this work?

Emotions, Health, and Illness

During the past three decades a new branch of medical science has developed called "psychoneuroimmunology." Scientists from several disciplines are studying the relationships between what happens in our external environment, how we interpret it psychologically, and how this in turn affects the body.

Our sense organs (eyes, ears, and so forth) perceive what is happening around us. Through special nerves they convey messages to specific parts of the brain—the centers for vision, hearing, touch, smell, or taste. From these centers, messages go to other parts of the nervous system, including those responsible for emotions. In those centers the sensations are interpreted and given meaning. What the person perceives as the meaning of an event stimulates an emotional response. It may be a response of happiness or grief, of peace or fear, of joy or anger, of envy, guilt, or shame. Whatever the response may be, it affects the heart and blood vessels, the digestive system, and other organs as well.

Our body has a system of glands that produce chemicals needed for different bodily processes. Certain glands produce chemicals we call hormones and put them directly into the blood. Hormones circulate in the blood stream, influencing our organs, and regulating basic bodily processes.

We now know that the brain is more than just a center for transmitting and receiving electrical messages through the nervous system to and from all parts of the body. The brain is also a gland, for it produces a variety of chemicals we call neuropeptides. These neuropeptides enter immediately into the blood and go throughout the body. They also influence our organs, each in a different way.

Our emotions influence the production of hormones by the glands and neuropeptides by the nervous system. A particular emotional state, such as joy, causes the production of certain neuropeptides. Other emotional states, such as jealousy, fear, or guilt, stimulate the production of other neuropeptides and hormones. Therefore, through the chemicals from our brain and glands, our emotions have definite effects on the functioning of our organs.

An Example: Effects of Long-term Stress

Several decades ago, Dr. Hans Selye of Toronto did extensive studies on the effects of stress on the body. He found that external and internal stress factors act on the adrenal glands. These glands produce hormones that help us respond to both physical and psychological trauma. A sudden fright will immediately increase our pulse rate and blood pressure. It will dilate the pupils of our eyes for better vision. It will divert blood flow away from the intestinal tract to the muscles. This is the so-called "flight response," a protective mechanism permitting a rapid physical response to a frightening experience. A sudden attack of anger produces a similar reaction that we could call a "fight response." These reactions result from the action of adrenaline on the heart, blood vessels, and other organs.[1]

Our bodies are well-equipped to handle sudden episodes of stress such as fear and anger. However, we are not well equipped to handle long-term, smoldering stress, physical or psychological. If we hold on to the fear, anger, or other negative emotions resulting from long-standing stress, they will cause the brain and glands to keep on producing the neuropeptides and hormones associated with them. These chemicals in turn will continue to act on our various organ systems which, over time, can become ill and produce symptoms of pain, indigestion, and weakness. The response to these chemicals can cause an increase in blood pressure, tension in certain muscles, and a variety of other physical problems.

It is clear that chronic stress of all sorts can be

harmful to our health. The stressors may be in the external environment—our circumstances. They may also be internal, coming from painful emotions, memories, and conflicts down in the subconscious mind. It is becoming increasingly clear that long-standing and poorly handled stress, whatever the cause or causes may be, can produce chronic inflammatory conditions. These include certain forms of arthritis, long-term skin disorders, and possibly even certain diseases of the nervous system. I believe Roger's hard, knobby, tender liver that I described in chapter 2 came, at least in part, from the chemicals produced as a result of the many stress factors in his life. Treatment of the symptoms and even of the inflammatory process of the disease usually fails to bring healing. Only as the causes of the stress, the negative feelings, and the destructive emotions are discovered and dealt with can real healing occur.

On a steaming hot day many years ago, I sat in a government office in the Congo trying to get official papers for our school of nursing. Sudden abdominal cramps signaled a bad case of diarrhea. Although this was my first episode of diarrhea in a long time, I immediately suspected the cause. The pressures of five years of stress-filled days and nights, with many frustrations along the way, had built up within me. My internal organs were now reacting to these pressures and, perhaps in a symbolic way, were attempting to rid my system of their effects. My diagnosis was correct, and the colitis symptoms persisted during the remaining four months of that term of service. They did not entirely subside until two months after we had left the field for a much-needed period of rest and restoration.

The good news is that positive (constructive, pleasurable) emotions cause our glands and brain to produce other hormones and neuropeptides. These have beneficial effects on our different organ systems, and they tend to promote health and increase our resistance to infections and other diseases.

Not Victims but Participants

This new understanding has brought about a remarkable change in our understanding of the healing arts. In former times, our medical forebears knew intuitively that tender loving care was important in speeding recovery, but they did not know why that was so. They supposed that the bodily response to infections, other diseases, and even negative events was "automatic," beyond conscious control. Now we are realizing that our physical response to events around us and to diseases that affect us is not altogether automatic.

We can exercise a certain measure of conscious control over what goes on in the chemistry of our bodies and the responses of our various organs. We can do this through changes in our thinking and emotions. We can replace negative emotions with positive ones, and we can change the ways we respond to our circumstances and to particular illnesses. In these ways we intervene in our own state of health and recovery from illness. We are not simply "victims" of our circumstances or of the diseases that can affect us. Rather, we can play an active role in how we respond to what happens to us.

We talk about this as a new development in medical science, but it is not really new. Three thousand years ago King Solomon stated the principle of psychoneuroimmunology in Proverbs 14:30: "Peace of mind makes the body healthy, but jealousy is like a cancer." What is new is that we are now discovering the mechanisms by which emotions affect the body. And this understanding enables us to better learn how we can intervene in these processes.

In the early 1970s, Norman Cousins published a book describing his remarkable recovery from a "fatal" illness. In 1964 Cousins, then editor of the *Saturday Review,* was stricken with a rapidly progressing and painful illness affecting his joints. There was no effective medical treatment for this illness, and Cousins's doctors told him that he did not have long to live. Cousins reasoned that allowing the probable fatal outcome of his illness to depress his spirit and his emotions would further cripple whatever physical defenses he had. If, on the other hand, he could fill his mind with positive, pleasurable emotions, this could perhaps strengthen his body's response to this destructive disease process. He took charge of his treatment and began reading amusing books and watching movie comedies. He discovered that ten minutes of genuine belly laughter could give him up to two hours of pain-free respite. Gradually his fever disappeared, the pain and weakness went away, and over a one-year period he returned to health. He spent the remaining two decades of his life working with medical scientists at UCLA to discover how hope and joy can strengthen health and help sick persons cope with illness.[2]

The heart and body function together. It appears that the heart actually rules over the body. How we think, how we feel, and how we look at life strongly influence our bodies. When we feel in control of our circumstances and are able to focus on what is positive, constructive, and joyful, our bodies respond with increased strength, and this promotes health. But frustration, depression, and negative emotions depress certain physiological functions and can diminish our health and our response to disease.

Our Defense against Diseases

One of our body's systems that is intimately connected to our thoughts and emotions is the immune system. This is the highly complex mechanism God created within us to protect our health and enable us to recover from illness.

Among the principal actors in our immune system are our white blood cells. They act like an internal army constantly prepared to fight against outside invaders—microbes in all their forms. They also act against inside disturbances, such as cells that become abnormal and that can eventually produce malignant tumors. One strain of white blood cells fights directly against many bacteria, surrounding and digesting them to eliminate them from our body. Other strains produce antibodies to specific microbes. These antibodies, which circulate in our blood, are biochemicals that attach to microbes, either preventing them from causing infections, or paralyzing them so that the white blood cells can eliminate them more easily.

Studies now show that the effectiveness of the whole immune system varies according to our emotional condition. Positive emotions tend to strengthen the immune system, enabling us to remain healthy and less susceptible to many diseases. When we are ill, positive emotions enable us to cope better with the disease. On the other hand, fear, anger, hatred, and other negative emotions tend to depress the immune system. During periods of stress we are much more likely to have colds, the flu, or other infections.[3]

The Disease-Immune System Balance

What actually happens when a serious infection occurs? Let's look at what happens when a person gets pneumonia, an infection that once had a high rate of mortality—and one that can still kill us. The invading bacteria of pneumonia attack the lungs, causing chest pain, a cough, and difficulty in breathing. They also produce poisons (toxins) that cause fever and other signs of the battle taking place in the body. These toxins likewise attack the immune system.

The immune system staggers briefly, and its strength is diminished. This permits the pneumonia bacteria to multiply rapidly in the body. However, the immune system mobilizes quickly to produce more white blood cells to attack the bacteria and to produce specific antibodies against them. Under normal circumstances, within a short period of time the antibodies immobilize the invading pneumonia organisms, thus facilitating the work of the white blood cells in destroying them. The level of immunity actually increases above normal, the number of bacteria decreases, and the tide of battle sways in the body's favor. Within a variable period of time, the white blood cells and antibodies gain the victory, and the person recovers from pneumonia.

The body's battle against infections
An infection brings into play what I call the disease/immune system balance. In this balance, two factors opposed to each other determine the outcome. The disease organisms—bacteria, viruses, or parasites—are on one side of the balance. The immune system—white blood cells, antibodies, and other complex elements—is on the other side. The victory is determined by the strength of the one as opposed to the other. Four factors determine the outcome of an infection.

The power, or virulence, of the invading organisms
The cold virus, pervasive as it is, is nevertheless a

rather weak virus and soon succumbs to our antibodies. Pneumonia bacteria are more virulent and can produce a serious infection. At the extreme end of the spectrum is the highly virulent Ebola virus that multiplies at an alarming speed, invades all of the body organs and tissues, and in most cases quickly leads to death.

The number of organisms that get into the body

If only a tiny number of organisms succeed in penetrating our tissues, our immune system can usually handle them quickly, and the infection will be aborted or abbreviated. If a large number penetrate the body, such as can occur with a large, dirty wound or a heavy exposure to someone else who has a serious infection, they present a major challenge to our defenses, and the outcome can be much more serious.

The strength of our own immune system

How prepared are we to cope with the infectious challenge? If our immune system is "battle ready" and our various defensive mechanisms are well-prepared, we can handle even a massive invasion of bacteria or viruses. But if our immune system has been weakened in any way, this tips the balance in favor of the infection. Inadequate nutrition, fatigue, or a high level of poorly handled stress can diminish the strength of the immune system and thus increase the risk of serious infections.

The quality and effectiveness of medicine

We have a whole spectrum of antibiotics to help us in the fight against bacterial infections. Antibiotics act against the invading bacteria to diminish their power. This makes the defensive action of the white blood cells easier, and it shortens the time of infection. Antibiotics have greatly changed the course of many infections and have saved the lives of multitudes of people who might otherwise have succumbed to overwhelming infection.

Unfortunately, we have no effective antibiotics to help us fight most viruses. For viral infections we are pretty much on our own. For colds, the flu, the various forms of hepatitis, shingles, and other viral infections, the body's protective processes are the principal and only real line of defense.

The body's battle against malignant diseases

How does the body defend itself against cancer, leukemia, and lymphomas that eat away the body from within? These diseases have the potential to lead to death.

We continue to find evidence that the immune system is much involved in protecting us from the development of malignancies and even in fighting against the malignant cells of cancer. One group of white blood cells has the specific role of identifying and destroying cells in the organs that have become abnormal and could become cancer cells. This type of white blood cell is called the "natural killer cell." These cells are the first line of protection against cancer.[4]

Most people don't realize that abnormal cells are constantly developing in our bodies. Potential cancers occur almost daily. Our killer cells, however, are always on guard, and they immediately destroy these abnormal or "rebellious" cells. If that is the case, why does cancer sometimes develop? As in the case of infections, the three key factors are: the number of abnormal cells that develop at one time, their potential strength, and the capacity of the immune system to handle them.

Serious Infection and a Troubled Heart

Ursula, a twenty-eight-year-old single woman from

Germany, was admitted to our hospital when she was very ill. She had developed symptoms of pneumonia three days before coming to us. Clinical examination and chest X-rays revealed a mycoplasma infection, a serious form of pneumonia that can also affect the heart. We immediately began intravenous antibiotics, but her condition grew worse and cardiac complications developed.

Ursula's sister, a nurse, had come with her, and she told us Ursula's story. Both girls had grown up in a Christian home, and their parents were very strict in their religious observances. As a young girl, Ursula was active in church, but during her high school years she lost interest in her faith. After high school she began working and became involved in activities contrary to her Christian upbringing and her parents' instructions. For ten years no one could talk to her about God or about faith.

As her condition worsened, Ursula refused to let anyone pray for her. Even the word "prayer" made her angry. When it seemed evident that she was dying, she called her sister to her and whispered, "I see my whole life and that I have wasted it. Do you think God can forgive me and accept me as his daughter?"

Her sister assured her that not only could God accept her but that God was waiting for her to come to him. She then heard Ursula whisper a prayer to God, asking for forgiveness and for him to please accept her into his kingdom. At her request, I prayed a simple prayer for her healing.

I sat with Ursula all through the long night. At midnight her pulse was very fast—160 beats per minute. Her lips were dusky blue, and she could breathe only sitting upright in bed. As the night progressed, her pulse and breathing gradually slowed, her color turned to pink, and by sun-up she was able to lie flat in bed. She awoke, smiled at her sister, and whispered, "I have found a new life." That afternoon she sat on the verandah with a guitar, singing songs of faith she had not sung for more than ten years.

What happened? A new insight into her life had come into Ursula's spirit. She was able to release the anger, bitterness, and rebellion in her heart and receive from God the peace for which she had been looking so desperately and unsuccessfully. Then her physiological defenses were quickly mobilized and, with the help of the medicines already in her body, she was able to overcome the infection. The healing of soul and spirit can have immense physiological effects.

There is another important lesson for us in this story. Antibiotics help us fight infections, but they do not cure us. We are cured by our own immune system—that array of white blood cells, antibodies, and other complex mechanisms that wage the real battle against the disease-producing organisms and eliminate them. Antibiotics help the body by attacking the invading organisms and damaging them in such a way as to enable the defensive mechanisms to get rid of them more quickly. It is our own body, however, that is the real victor. We gave Ursula effective antibiotics for her pneumonia, but they did not cure her, nor could they. It was only when her heart had been healed that her immune system switched back on and she was able to recover.[5]

I have described some powerful examples of how the heart affects health and healing. Now we must look at it in more detail. Understanding what is in the center of our life is of great importance in enabling us to live healthy lives and, when the need arises, to cope with illness.

5

The Architecture of the Heart

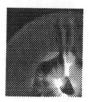

In chapter four of the book of Proverbs, we read, "My child, pay attention to what I say. Listen to my words. Never let them get away from you. Remember them and keep them in your heart. They will give life and health to anyone who understands them. Be careful how you think; your life is shaped by your thoughts" (Proverbs 4:20-23).

Jesus recognized the importance of the heart in the life of a person. He said that evil things in the heart pollute the whole person and result in all kinds of destructive actions (Mark 7:21-23). The heart, therefore, is a very important place. It is the center of our life and determines who we are, what we do, and how we live in this world. It has an immense influence on our health.

All of us struggle with personal problems, and the seat of those problems is in the heart. Dr. Paul Tournier, a wise physician of the whole person, wrote in Switzerland in 1964 that our struggles with these problems—conflicts, rebellions, negative attitudes, moral failings, and spiritual anxieties—have a considerable influence on our health.[1] It follows from this that the healing of the heart—replacing the negative with the positive—can prevent certain illnesses and can reinforce the body when it must cope with disease. Before we can consider the healing of the heart, we must understand what it is. What is inside us that makes us who we are?

A Simple—but Effective—Example

As I worked with many sick persons and also taught young physicians and nursing students, I realized that the term "heart" was an abstract concept and difficult to comprehend. I looked for some way to make this concept more concrete. So I have compared the heart to a home (figures 1 and 2). We have used this image to help physicians, nurses, and pastors better comprehend how to help sick persons. We have the image in figure 2 on the wall of our consulting rooms to help sick persons grasp what is going on inside them.

The comparison of a heart to a home is admittedly simplistic. The way our inner life works is quite complex, as any student of psychology knows. We can't extend the allegory of a home any further than the brief explanations in this chapter. Nevertheless, this simple design has proved to be most helpful both as a teaching instrument and as an aid in counseling.

The symbol of the heart as our home is useful for self-examination. A personal inventory can be a helpful exercise for someone who is ill or who is aware of deep-seated problems. I have used it many times myself when I have been ill or have been trying to work through stresses in my life.

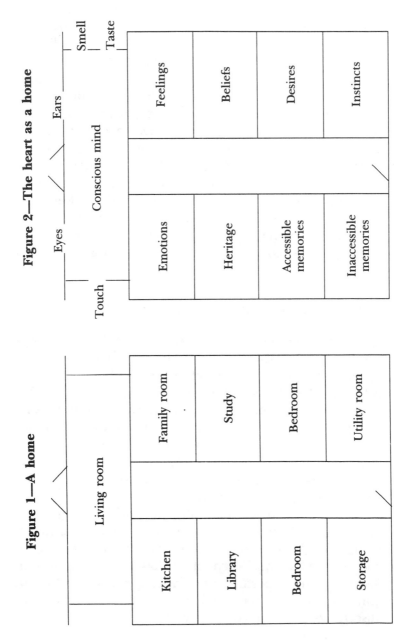

Figure 1—A home

Living room		
Kitchen		Family room
Library		Study
Bedroom		Bedroom
Storage		Utility room

Figure 2—The heart as a home

Eyes · Ears · Smell · Taste · Touch

Conscious mind

Emotions		Feelings
Heritage		Beliefs
Accessible memories		Desires
Inaccessible memories		Instincts

The heart is not a quiet, tranquil place. It is a collection of rooms—places within us—that are buzzing with communications coming and going. Its walls resound with many emotions, thoughts, memories, and instincts that travel from one room to another and slip in and out of doors and windows. Outside the house of our heart is the outside world that is our body. Messages from the heart travel constantly to all parts of the body, receiving an abundance of sensations and coordinating a multitude of activities.

When there is internal harmony and consistency, the whole person can function well. But when one part is overstressed, disturbed, or ill, or when conflicts occur between the areas of the heart and between the heart and the body, functional effectiveness (health) is impaired and illness can result.

The Living Room: Our Conscious Mind

The living room is the entrance to the home; it represents the conscious mind. This is where we think, reflect, and form our opinions. It is the seat of the intellect, the reason, and also the imagination. It actually is a very small room, for we can only think one thought at a time. Yet in all our waking moments, the living room is where we are. The furniture, the paintings on the wall, and perhaps the flowers on the table symbolize the thoughts we enjoy or the things that can clutter our thoughts.

A wide door opens out into the world and gives access to it. Through this door we express what is in our mind. We do it by our actions, by our speech, and by the non-verbal ways each of us has of expressing ourselves: gestures, posture, and facial expressions. No one can see into our conscious mind. However, others can discern some of the contents by what we say and do.

The windows in the living room let the lights and sounds of the outside world into the house. The windows represent the five senses through which we perceive what is going on around us. Through our sight, hearing, touch, taste, and smell we become conscious of what is happening in our immediate environment.

The conscious mind is where we make decisions or judgments. We sometimes call this our conscience, that part of our personality that decides whether something is right or wrong, or whether it is good or bad for us.

The Subconscious Mind

All that is beyond the living room is the subconscious mind. This is a very big place, for we keep a great many things here. A hall runs from the living room to the back of the house. The various rooms connect with each other and with the conscious mind through the hall. Let's go through each of these rooms.

The kitchen: our emotions

One of the principal rooms in the home is the kitchen. We keep our emotions here, for emotions occupy an important place in our heart. This is where we laugh or cry, where we joke or get angry with each other.

An emotion is an internal response to an external event, a strong psychic energy that influences the body as well as the rest of the mind. What comes into the mind through the windows of the senses stays not only in the thoughts in the living room but passes quickly into the room of the emotions as well. As we saw in the last chapter, each type of emotional response "cooks" up a batch of neuropeptides. These circulate immediately, not only to the other rooms in the heart but also to the organs in our body, and they influence organ activity. Our emotional "kitchen" affects every aspect of our life.

There is much movement into and out of this room. Events from the outside stimulate the emotions, and the emotions strongly influence our thoughts, expressions, and behavior. It is in the emotions that the heart discerns the meaning of each event and what the response to that event should be. Imagine yourself sitting around the kitchen table with your feelings, desires, beliefs, and intuition. You are discussing the meaning of what is going on in the world around you and how you should respond to it. This response often is in imperative terms. If the emotional energy of your response is powerful, like that which occurs in sudden anger or fear, an abrupt outburst of emotions can go straight through the living room and out the front door before the conscious mind can check it. You can speak angry words without thinking, or lash out at someone before taking stock of what would be appropriate.

On the other hand, the energy of strong emotions needs to be diffused in one way or another. A strong-willed person may keep inside even intense emotions and not allow them out through speech or other forms of expression. Bottled-up emotional energy can manifest itself in ways detrimental to health, even to physical health. If the judgment decides that a particular emotion cannot be expressed, then ways need to be found to use that energy in constructive ways. The events stimulating that emotional energy need to be reinterpreted so as to diminish or dissipate that energy in constructive ways.

If negative emotions such as anger, fear, shame, or envy are kept pent-up in the subconscious mind for a long time, they will continue to stimulate the production of neuropeptides that act on blood pressure, the digestion, and other organs and systems in the body. Chronic production of these neuropeptides by negative emotions may eventually result in a physical or psychological illness. Imagine the effect in your real home of allowing a bunch of rotten eggs to simmer slowly on the stove for many days. Phew! It would turn your stomach. In reality, this is exactly what simmering anger or bitterness does. If untreated (not cleaned up), it may even poke a hole in your stomach. We call this a "perforated stomach ulcer."

Mrs. Katanda came frequently to the hospital with acute attacks of asthma. One day, when her symptoms had improved, I talked to her about her life. Her husband frequently abused her verbally. Their five children were often screaming at each other and at her. As these external tensions mounted around her, they triggered intense anger in her heart and precipitated an acute asthmatic attack. In other words, external tensions stimulated anger in her heart. The chemicals produced in response to the anger caused tension and spasms in the muscles lining her breathing tubes, and an asthma attack would result. Providing relief was our immediate concern. Helping her find solutions to the external problems and to her response of anger became a long-term concern. Emotions can affect many of our internal organs.

The family room: our feelings

Across the hall is the family room, the room where we keep our feelings. How do feelings differ from emotions? They differ more in degree than in kind. Emotions are like a hot fire with flames leaping up. By contrast, feelings are like warm glowing coals that persist even when there are not flames. Feelings are the impressions we have about ourselves, the world around us, and the circumstances in which we find ourselves. If we perceive our circumstances to be good, we feel happy, comfortable, and secure. If not, we may feel uncertain, insecure, and uncomfortable.

Our attitudes, our sentiments, and our intuition are in this room. It is hard to distinguish between feelings, attitudes, sentiments, and intuition, and it is not necessary. They have to do with our orientation toward a particular aspect of our lives, how we feel about something. Often feelings do not break out into the living room, our conscious thoughts. Nevertheless, we sense an inner impression down inside that something attracts us or else make us uneasy.

The study: our beliefs and values
Beyond the family room is the study, a room where we reflect on life and the world around us. This is where we keep our beliefs. We keep much more than just religious beliefs in this room. Our beliefs about everything are there—what we accept as true about any and all areas of our lives. We have beliefs about our family, our work, our community, and our nation. We have beliefs about fun and pleasure, about death and dying, and about the life we have been given. We have strong beliefs about sexuality, and particular beliefs about our own personal gender.

Imagine a big desk in this room surrounded by shelves that are stacked with labeled files: God; Family; Marriage; Sports; Politics; Religion; My Work; Food; Recreation; Men; Women; Honesty; Money. . . . We can pull down a file at will, add to it, or make changes in what it contains.

Here also is where we store our values. We keep our values as we keep books—arranged on shelves by subject matter. Much of our behavior comes from what we believe is good and valuable for us. We do what we do in order to gain approval and to avoid conflict, failure, and shame. We guard this room carefully, admitting new beliefs and values reluctantly and changing beliefs or values only with great difficulty. As we grow and learn more, we change some of them and acquire new ones from our experience. It is important to examine our beliefs carefully and to try to understand what we believe. Our beliefs affect how we think, the way we perceive our world, and, ultimately, how we act.

The library: our heritage

Across the hall from the study is the library, with book-lined shelves, a study table, and comfortable chairs. Here we keep the heritage we have received from previous generations. There is evidence that a deep part of our personality comes from this heritage. Our parents, our ancestors, and our culture pass on to us the view of life into which we were born. We guard all this in the many books on the shelves lining the wall.

This heritage greatly affects how we think, how we feel, and how we respond to the world around us. It acts within us as a strong brake on any major change in our lives. We may not understand our deep resistance to change, but the source is in what has been passed on to us from the generations before us.

The bedroom: our desires

Further down the hall are bedrooms. In one of these bedrooms we keep our desires and our drives for power, for wealth, for pleasure, and for sexual satisfaction. We have desires for the approval of others, for prestige and glory, and also the desire to avoid shame. We likewise have a strong drive for creativity, to bring into being something that is somehow a unique expression of self. The drive for learning—for gaining new knowledge or acquiring new skills—resides in this bedroom. We may also have a drive for spiritual knowledge—for knowing the truth and for knowing God.

The storeroom and second bedroom: our memories
Every event that has ever occurred in our lives, from the day we were born until this present moment, is recorded in the memory and stored in the subconscious mind. Some of these memories we can recall, and they are in another bedroom. However, the vast bulk of our memories is lost to recall, and we keep them in a large storeroom at the end of the hall or in the attic or basement.

Imagine these rooms filled with filing cabinets reaching to the ceiling. Each of the many drawers is filled with separate folders where we file the memory of each event. In the memory bedroom are those that are easy to recall. We can quickly retrieve them and bring them into the thoughts of our conscious mind. Some of the retrievable memories may date back to early childhood. They remain vivid because they are memories of important and significant events, and they are available for recall to the conscious mind. These filing cabinets are in good condition and the drawers open easily, although some open more easily than others.

The unavailable memories are lost to conscious recall. We can imagine that the drawers of these filing cabinets are rusted shut, or are locked and the keys are lost. Memories from infancy and early childhood and a multitude of memories during our growing-up years are among those lost to recall. Other memories, even of recent events, are lost because they were filed in disorder, or else because the event was not vivid or important enough to merit being classified in a retrievable place.

What is important to understand is that every memory, retrievable or not, continues to influence what goes on in our minds. The memories of birth are almost universally lost to conscious recall. Nevertheless, although they are buried in a rusty filing drawer, they can continue to influence feelings, emotions, and intuition. It is possible that even perceptions "in utero," from before birth, may be hidden away in file drawers in a dark corner in the attic or the basement and still have an influence on our current lives. Memories of difficulties before birth, or of trauma during or immediately after birth can have long-lasting effects on mental and even physical health.

The utility room: our instincts

Every home has some sort of utility room for the heating unit, the air-conditioner, the laundry facilities, and food storage. The heat and the air are connected to every room of the house through big vents that carry the warm or cool air throughout the house. We can compare this utility room to our instincts.

Instincts are the deep-seated, almost automatic response of the mind related to the fundamental needs of life. They are for our immediate protection, for the preservation of life, and for the defense of our health. We rarely give them any thought. Rather, we automatically do what is necessary to protect ourselves, to avoid injury, and to assure our basic needs for air, water, and food.

Instincts are powerful. With our conscious minds, even with great determination, we can seldom override them. No one can commit suicide by deciding not to breathe; the instinct for air soon overrides any conscious determination to refuse air into the lungs. It is possible to starve oneself to death, but even that requires great mental effort.

Spirit

In what room can we assign our spirit? Our spirit, as I understand it, pervades all the rooms, including that of the conscious mind. It is the very center of our being and has access to all areas of the mind. As I wrestle with the deep questions of my life, I think. But I also feel, I intuit, and I delve into my memories of past experiences. My emotions become involved as well as my beliefs and my drives. If I set about consciously to do as Socrates recommended to all his students: "Know thyself," my whole being becomes involved. My spirit is me, my whole self, trying to understand better who I am and why I am here.

In the same way, as I talk to God and try to listen to him, this involves my thoughts. It usually involves my feelings, my intuition, and the deeper levels of my heart. An impression comes, or a deep feeling that something is right or that something else is not right. If the impression I receive from God is strong, it may stir my emotions, bringing joy or even tears. It is with my whole self that I come before the Lord, the Maker of heaven and earth.

Interconnections

Many interactions occur between the various areas of our heart. The impressions we receive through our senses come first into the conscious mind and then enter the various rooms in the subconscious mind. They are filed in a memory drawer in the memory bedroom, and many of them will eventually be transferred into another drawer in the storeroom at the back of the home. The events we experience stimulate the emotions and influence the desires and drives.

In the same way, what is in the subconscious mind can come into the conscious mind and influence it. Some emotions or desires enter quietly; others may burst violently into the conscious mind and even out through the door of expression to the outside world. We often find ourselves doing or saying things with little or no thought, and then we wonder why we have done them. Even during sleep, the subconscious mind remains active, and our dreams are the processing of present and past symbols and events.

The Back Door

Somewhere in the depths of our heart is one other feature of our home: the back door. This is the door to our spiritual environment, and it opens from the inside. Through this door we can reach outward to make contact with the spiritual world—with God or with other spiritual powers. Prayer to God is communication through this door, speaking to him and listening for his responses. He can communicate with us by means of new thoughts, strong impressions, dreams, visions, or through words spoken by others. Other spiritual powers of good or of evil can likewise communicate with us through this door if we wish to hear them. It is through this door that we can invite Christ to come into our heart. Or, if we wish, we can invite other spirits to come in. We must guard this door closely, for our relation with the spiritual world strongly influences our spiritual, psychological, and even physical health.

Hygiene of the Heart

Guarding the heart is essential for our health. What we allow to enter our mind and heart will be a part of our personality for the remainder of our lives and can affect us for good or for ill. What takes place in the inner recesses of our being, much of which may never come into conscious thought, can strengthen or weaken our tissues, our organs, and our immune system.

While we cannot avoid every painful and frightening experience in our lives, it is important to our psychological and physical well-being to make good judgments when we *can* control what we see, hear, and perceive through our senses. Those of us who are parents need to help our children discern what is good to allow into their minds and hearts—and also what is harmful and what should be kept out.

A couple of years ago, our neighbors received a video of a well-known film of high regard and they invited us over to see it. About twenty minutes into the film, my spirit revolted. I knew the theme of the movie was supposed to be positive, showing how a courageous man risked his life and career to help others. Yet I did not want to store in the file drawers of my memory those horrible scenes of killing, of blood oozing from brains, and of explicit sexual behavior. So I made the decision to reject this, and I left and went home. I asked the Lord to wash away those images, and I consciously tried to forget them.

The Apostle Paul counsels us to fill our minds with what is good, true, noble, right, pure, lovely, honorable, and worthy of praise (Philippians 4:8). That, by the way, is marvelous psychology and very good for one's health. As Jesus said in Mark 7, it is from the heart that evil thoughts and desires come. The conscious mind can act as a filter. The images that come from the memory or emotions can be evaluated. Those that seem good can be reinforced, and those that seem evil or sinful can be rejected. As we will see later, many evil memories and feelings can be healed.

6

What's Sin Got to Do with It?

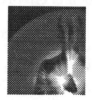

W e've talked about *how* we get sick—the physical processes and how they are affected by our emotions and other factors. But none of those explanations answers the more fundamental question: Why do we have the capacity to get sick in the first place? Where did illness and disease begin? How can we reconcile their presence in the world with our faith in a loving God?

The Biblical Perspective

In the third chapter of Genesis, the Bible declares that disease and death entered human life when our ancestors sinned. The word "sin" makes us uncomfortable. But sin is more than just a religious word; it is a word that applies to every aspect of human life. It describes our condition, regardless of our beliefs or practices.

Most cultures of the world, including the ancient Hebrew culture of the Bible, believe there is a close relationship between sin and sickness. It is our modern Western culture that cannot accept that belief. But we aren't comfortable with our denial of it. Dr. Karl Menninger, an eminent psychiatrist, wrote a book about this entitled, *Whatever Happened to Sin?*[1] In reality, that is not the question, for nothing has happened to sin. It remains as powerful as ever. It is we who have changed. We would like to believe that disease is just a physical phenomenon that happens to us and has nothing to do with how we live, think, feel, or relate to one another. Nothing could be further from the truth.

The story of the origin of sin is in the second and third chapters of the book of Genesis. Sin is a rejection of God. It is a rebellion against what it true. God created us to live in harmonious relationships with each other, with him, and with the physical world. Sin hurts or breaks these relationships, and thus it leads to alienation. When our ancestors sinned, they threw out the "manufacturer's instructions," the way of life God carefully laid out for them to follow. They had a high-sounding reason to do so—they wanted to be free. But the result of their rebellion was that they lost the authority over the world that God had given them. They also defaced the image of God that he had stamped within them. All of this has a lot to do with health and healing, and much to do with illness and death.

In Genesis chapter 2 we read that God planted in the Garden of Eden a tree whose fruit gives knowledge of what is good and what is evil. He forbade our ancestors to eat the fruit of that tree, warning them that if they did so they would die. It will remain a mystery why God gave humankind such a choice. We can make all kinds of speculations—and theologians have been doing so for centuries—but it is doubtful that any "reason" we can think of will fully satisfy us.

God certainly knew the enormity of evil and its destructive power; God knew the disorder and disasters that would come from our human freedom to choose evil. How can we reconcile this with our belief in the goodness of God? We cannot do so completely, but in faith we can hold onto the goodness of God, believing that somehow the goodness of our freedom surpasses the magnitude of the evil in which we are living. Goodness is eternal because it is part of the nature of God and as such is part of our own nature. Evil is historical, not eternal, and one day it will pass away.

The Genesis story provides a clear picture of our problem; we rejected our relationship with God, and we rejected the world as it was given to us. We sinned (and continue to sin) out of our choice to live independently of the God who made us. We may still pretend that we love God, worship God, and are doing what God wants by doing good things. However, we are doing it on our own terms rather than on God's terms and in obedience to his instruction. All of us stand condemned on this account.

By choosing spiritual autonomy, Adam and Eve brought evil into human history, and transmitted the bent toward evil to us. In doing so, they failed to grasp what God had clearly indicated to them. We are free to make choices, but we are not free to choose the consequences of those choices. God had told them, "The day you eat of the fruit of that tree, you will surely die." They were free to eat it, or not to eat it, but they were not free to avoid the death that would ensue if they did. We also are free to make choices, but we are not free to reject the consequences of those choices.

We find in Genesis chapter 3 the consequences of Adam and Eve's choice. By rejecting God's plan for order and harmony in life, our ancestors introduced disorder into human life. The disorder spread to all aspects of life, disrupted all relationships, and brought with it the disease, natural disasters, and death that continue to this day.

Our Relationship with God—Spiritual Death

God created us to live in relationship with him and to be dependent on him. He put within our hearts a deep desire to live in union with him, to be in communication with him, and to conform to his purpose and plan for us. When our ancestors disobeyed their Maker, this relationship was broken by their own choice. They rejected God and became alienated from him who is the source of all life.

St. Augustine said, "Thou hast created us for Thyself, and our hearts are restless until they find their rest in Thee."[2] This is to say that God made us with a hole in the heart that only he can fill. When we threw God out, our hearts shrank as that hole collapsed. Only God can refill it and expand our hearts. If we have not allowed God to fill this hole, we are strongly impelled to try to fill it in other ways, and some of them may seriously harm our life and our health.

Our Relationship with Self—Sickness of the Soul

This first sin deeply disturbed a person's relationship with the self. Immediately after disobeying God, Adam and Eve turned their eyes back on themselves, and they perceived something was wrong. They saw they were naked, exposed, stripped of their joyful harmony with the world, with each other, and with God. Self-affirmation, the joy of living, and the assurance of having a place to be somebody of value were gone. A flood of negative emotions inundated their hearts—shame, fear, guilt. Because of all of this, Adam and Eve did two things: they tried to cover their nakedness, and they went into hiding. Sin leads to self-alienation.

Our Relationships with Others—Social Disorder

When Adam and Eve sinned, social disorder began immediately. This was inevitable because our ancestors now became self-oriented persons. Instead of living under the rule of God's Spirit and in harmony with all of God's creatures, each person became independent, thinking primarily of himself or of herself.

Gender conflict began in the Garden. Soon brother-to-brother and parent-child conflicts began, and society quickly became a tangle of people in conflict with one another. Each person and group was primarily concerned for its own interests and how to protect and expand those interests, often at the expense of others. The human heart became infected by the desire to control others. This led to the breakdown of trust and the suspicion that others might be trying to dominate and even destroy us. The resulting social disorder has led to wars, displacements, and the exploitation of the powerless by the powerful, all of which diminishes or destroys the health of millions of people.

Our Relationship with the Natural World—Loss of Dominion

The authority God gave our ancestors over the created world was disrupted by the Fall. Instead of exercising a wise God-oriented control over nature, we are subject to the greater forces of nature and are often victims of its power. The decreased fertility and diminished productivity of the soil in many places in the world are consequences of the disorder we brought into the world. The individual and corporate sins of greed and the desire for excessive profits have resulted in the pollution of the air, soil, and water. The health of us all suffers from the evil we are doing to the environment.

Lost Sense of Responsibility

When our ancestors rebelled against God, a fundamental change occurred at the very center of their personalities. Instead of admitting wrong-doing and accepting responsibility for their actions, they tried to turn the responsibility back to God. Adam sinned, then blamed his companion. He also blamed God who had given him this companion. Eve sinned and blamed the serpent. Each one said, in effect, "It's not my fault." In so doing, our ancestors turned from being active co-managers with God of their lives, to being passive victims of what other spiritual or physical forces inflicted on them. Thus began the tendency to shrug the responsibility for our own lives and actions.

From this we see—in a very general sense—how sin introduced disorder, disease, and death into human life. Instead of being concerned with our relationship with God and with the interests of others, we became preoccupied with ourselves.

Sin is vastly more than just a psychological problem. It is a potent spiritual power in the world. Hatred is real and destructive. Millions of Jews were destroyed in the gas chambers of Nazi Germany not just because hatred is psychological but because it is a real—and spiritual—power. It continues to destroy millions today—in central Africa, in parts of Europe and the Middle East, and on the streets of many of our own cities and towns. Hatred takes hold of a person's psyche, and that hold is immensely powerful and real. It requires a greater power to overcome it, and that power has come from Jesus Christ. Before we consider what Christ has done to help us, we must see how sin works in us on a personal basis and how sickness can result from it.

Does God Want Us to Be Sick or to Be Healthy?

I have based my life and my professional career on the premise that God wants us to be healthy. I believe this is what the Bible teaches us, and medical science is likewise committed to this premise. Here are three reasons I believe God wants us to have health.

1. Disease and death were not part of Eden. The account of the Garden of Eden is very brief, but there are sufficient reasons to conclude that disease, disasters, and death were not part of the Edenic life of Adam and Eve. Were there mosquitoes in the Garden? Was the tuberculosis bacillus there, or viruses, or the streptococcus germ? Obviously we do not know, but it is safe to assume that, even if they were there, they did not affect Adam and Eve. That would have been contrary to God's original plan of life for them, a plan for life and not for death, for health and not for illness.

2. Jesus, God's Son, came to do the will of his Father and to accomplish the work God sent him

to do. A primary focus of Jesus' ministry on earth was healing sick people. If God wanted us to be sick, why did he send his Son to heal the sick? And why did his Son then tell us to do the same thing?

3. There will be no suffering, crying, or pain in heaven (Revelation 21:4). In heaven we will experience the perfect relationship with God that he intended in the beginning. God promises that this eternal life will be free of pain and illness.

To help us lead healthy and productive lives, God gave us laws, regulations, and guidelines regarding our behaviors and our inner life. Their purpose is not to confine or inhibit us. Rather they are to guide our living so that we can approach the abundant life Jesus offers and maximize our creative possibilities.

Sickness and Sin?

If original sin led to illness, disorder, and death in the world, then does that mean that when I become ill, it's because I have sinned? We must be very careful here. There is more than one answer to this question.

Personal sin can have a physical effect on us

Specific sins can in fact lead to certain illnesses and diseases. Sexually transmitted diseases are an obvious example. Habits of poor hygiene or of faulty nutrition open the door to many diseases. We are well aware of the links between habits of addiction and the diseases they can cause. We are not as conscious of how attitudinal habits of high stress and of frequent interpersonal confrontations can damage our organ systems, but these problems are real, widespread in society, and can actually lead to death.

According to the biblical account, certain habits and behavior patterns—deception, the exploitation of other people, and sexual promiscuity, among others— are sinful. They destroy relationships, can harm other people, and are outward manifestations of an inner rebellion against God's plan for our lives. Often these habits and behavior patterns lead to illness. In these cases there is a direct link between sin as rebellion, sinful behavior as a manifestation of this rebellion, and illness.

Personal sin can have a psychological effect on us

Holding onto destructive emotions such as anger, jealousy, or hatred (sinful because when we hold onto them, they harm or destroy relationships) can either cause certain stress-related illnesses or else weaken the immune system and thus allow a disease to develop. They can act on other organs in the body to cause disturbances such as increased blood pressure, an elevated level of cholesterol, spasms of muscles in organs such as the lungs or the intestines, or inflammation in other tissues. In this case, we can say that sinful thoughts, emotions, or behaviors act as predisposing factors that can lead to illness.

In addition, unhealthy attitudes when we are ill can impede recovery and even aggravate the illness.

Other people's sins can lead to our illness

We must also recognize that much illness comes, not because of personal sin but as a result of the sins of others.

A mission executive whom we will call John visited leaders of a partner church in a Central American country. One of the leaders of the partner church seemed somewhat distracted. He told John that his sixteen-year-old daughter, Sylvia, had been suffering from severe and painful menstrual bleeding for a year. He asked John if he would be willing to go with him to his home and pray with her.

Later in the afternoon John went with this leader to his tiny home along with eight deacons from the church. After a short discussion of the problem, the father led the group into the small bedroom where Sylvia was lying on the bed, obviously in pain. As John bent down to put his hand on the young woman's head, the eight deacons knelt in a circle around the bed. John prayed in English for Sylvia, asking the Lord to comfort her, to take away her pain, and to heal her in his good time. When he had finished praying, she smiled weakly and thanked John and the others in Spanish for their concern and prayer.

A month later John received a letter telling him about Sylvia's situation. A few days after the group had prayed for Sylvia, she had called her father and told him the secret that was weighing so heavily upon her. A year previously, she had been sexually abused by a leader in the theological school of the church, a man who was a close friend of her father. Because of that relationship and the responsibility this man had in teaching young pastors, Sylvia hadn't been able to reveal what had happened. From the day of that traumatic abuse, Sylvia had bled and been in constant pain. However, something in her heart was released when John and the deacons prayed with her, even though she did not understand the prayer with her mind. She finally was able to confide in her father and tell him the whole story. Appropriate action was taken by the church leaders in regard to the guilty leader, and further prayer with Sylvia resulted in complete healing of her pain and bleeding.

In a more general sense, corporate sins affect the health of most of us. This includes the dumping of industrial wastes that puts toxic products in the soil or water, atmospheric pollution, and paying employees less than a living wage. The corporate sins of systemic violence and warfare have reached tragic proportions and are sacrificing the lives and health of millions of people.

Sometimes there is no clear relationship between sin and sickness

In many cases, there seem to be no sinful behaviors involved. Even here, however, a bit of introspection can be helpful. How am I responding to this illness? If I dwell on thoughts and feelings of bitterness, or let anger toward others or God fester, or refuse to respond positively to the situation, I am harming myself.

Two Words of Caution

First, can the knowledge that I have messed up areas of my life increase my guilt and thus further depress my immune system? Of course it can. But that knowledge can also lead me to seek healing. There is a solution for guilt, and we will come to that solution in the next chapter. I can be like Adam and Eve, blaming someone else or even God himself for all these unhealthy things in my heart. Or else I can deal with these problems and bring them to the feet of Jesus Christ, who can remove them and heal me. The choice is mine.

Second, who can accuse sick persons of having committed sin and therefore of having brought their illness on themselves? Can health professionals, or pastoral counselors, or even close family members point the finger of accusation? Absolutely not. When a person is ill, only one person in all the world should raise the question of sin, and that is the sick person. Let me illustrate this by a personal example.

Sometime around 1980 the virus of hepatitis B entered my body without causing immediate illness. A routine physical examination in 1982 discovered it. In retrospect, I probably came into contact with it in the surgical theater because many persons on whom I operated in our hospital in the Congo had the virus. My diagnosis in 1982 was chronic active hepatitis, and I was counseled to "take it easy." However, in the pressure-filled environment of a big mission hospital, trying to cope with enormous needs with few personnel and limited resources, I felt that taking it easy was not possible for me. By early 1987 the inflammation in my liver had progressed to the point of early cirrhosis. My energy level had diminished, and I knew I was ill.

A month prior to our departure on a long-overdue sabbatical leave, I was leading a seminar on community health with leaders from several villages. We were discussing the Old Testament principles of health and how our disobedience to God's laws had brought disorder and disease into our lives. We also saw how obedience to God's commandments could restore some order and a measure of health to ourselves and to our communities. I told the participants to consider the Ten Commandments in Exodus 20, asking them, "Which of those commandments influence our health?"

The usual response to this question is the seventh commandment: You shall not commit adultery. To my surprise, a schoolteacher replied immediately, "The fourth commandment—Remember the Sabbath day to keep it holy." He explained that if we do not rest one day a week and take care of our bodies, we can become ill.

Those words resounded like a thunderclap in my heart. This man had unwittingly pointed out my sin to me. *I* was the one who had not respected the Sabbath, who had not cared for the body God had given me. *I* had sinned by working seven days a week, justifying it on the basis that I was "doing God's work." Many Sundays I would say to myself, "I'll worship God in the operating room." Hence the inflammation of my liver was progressing. Oh yes, I loved God and I was giving my life for him. I was "doing his will" by serving others seven days a week. I was "glorifying him" by caring for many sick people and curing some of them "in Jesus' name." But it was on my own terms, not God's. Now God was showing me my sin.

This schoolteacher, of course, had not accused me of sin. It was the Spirit of God who accused me. He took this man's words and made them penetrate my heart, showing me I was sinning by abusing the body God had given me. As the animated discussion swirled around me, I bowed my spirit before the Almighty Father, confessed my sin, and asked for forgiveness. That was the beginning of my healing. But more about that later on.

We see then that an intimate though complex relationship exists between sin and sickness. My hepatitis B was a disease that came to me "in the line of duty" through no conscious sin of my own. But my illness— that is, my response to the hepatitis infection—was intermingled with attitudes and behavior that were sinful and that hindered the recuperative powers of my body.

Illnesses of the Heart

Now let us go back to our image of the heart and see the problems and illnesses that occur as disorder comes into the many "rooms" within us. The disorder may be the result of personal sin or of the sin of someone else. On the other hand, it may have no direct link with sin at all, coming simply from the general disorder of the marred world in which we live. Awareness of disorder in the heart is the beginning of our restoration.

Emotions

Retained anger, envy, jealousy, and hatred for another person are sinful emotions. The events that produced these emotions may have been beyond our control, but our reaction to them is within our control. Jesus said, "Whoever is angry with his brother will be brought to trial" (Matthew 5:22). To what trial? I believe it is to the trials of self-inflicted illness, for these retained destructive emotions can have powerful disease-producing effects on the body: headaches, intestinal spasms, high blood pressure, or stomach disorders.

Many who suffer from chronic pains or inflammatory syndromes have deeply buried anger in their hearts against parents or other significant persons. This anger may now be totally repressed, yet it is there and it "eats" the connective tissue, the joint membranes, or the intestinal lining. The sin of an unforgiving spirit is extremely dangerous for our physical health.

A sense of guilt seriously interferes with meaningful, creative activity. It erodes the power to concentrate, and it can lead to depression. So can shame or a sense of rejection. At the same time, physical symptoms can develop, with one or more organs unable to function in equilibrium with the others. The immune system can be depressed by these unhealthy feelings, thus diminishing the power to resist infections. Fre-

quent colds, episodes of the flu, or other types of repeated infections may reflect unresolved problems
buried in the feelings.

Are fear, shame, and a sense of rejection sinful?
These feelings come to all of us, and are morally neu-
tral. How we handle them or fail to handle them is
important and this brings in moral considerations. If
we fail to handle these feelings properly, not only do
we become morally culpable but we may also become
sick.

Desires and drives
This area of our hearts is especially susceptible to sin
and to unhealthy influences. Greed and covetousness
are sinful and can be very deleterious to health. The
constant desire to have what others have, to surpass
our neighbors in prestige, to accumulate possessions
simply for the satisfaction of having much—this can
lead to physical illness. Such desires are sinful because
they are self-oriented. They reject open constructive
relationships with others and lead to unrighteous and
unhealthy rivalries.

Uncontrolled desires for money, for sexual pleasure,
and for power over others are sinful because they
make us seek our satisfaction from something or
someone other than God. Such unchecked desires
quickly disrupt social relationships—in many cases
damaging other people—thus stimulating a variety of
unhealthy emotions. In this way they can destabilize
normal healthy physiology and lead to the dysfunc-
tioning of organs or to chronic painful processes in
various parts of the body.

Beliefs
Conflicting beliefs can have serious consequences on
mental and even physical health. A fascinating story

from the third and fourth chapters of the Old Testament book of Daniel illustrates this.

King Nebuchadnezzar was one of the remarkable rulers in world history. On one occasion he had an enormous idol built and commanded all the people of his empire to worship that idol. Three men from Israel courageously refused to worship that idol, and the king had them thrown into a fiery furnace. God delivered the three men from the flames, and Nebuchadnezzar was immensely impressed. He recognized the superior power of the God of Israel and made a decree that no one throughout his whole kingdom could speak disrespectfully of this powerful God of Israel. He added the God of Israel to the collection of gods in his heart. However, when he had signed and sealed this decree, he went back out to fall down and worship his idol.

Nebuchadnezzar's heart became divided between his idol and what he had observed of the power of God. A year later he became psychotic, or as the Bible describes it, "as a wild beast." He remained that way for seven years, driven from the presence of other people, until he was able to resolve the conflict in his heart and recognize there is only one God. Changing one belief for another (conversion) can be healthy, but allowing conflicting beliefs to co-exist in the heart can destroy inner peace. A divided heart can lead to mental breakdown and sometimes to physical disease.

For this reason involvement in occult beliefs and practices can be dangerous, especially if we try to combine them with the Christian faith. Occult beliefs pull a person in one direction while Christian beliefs and values pull in the opposite direction. The result can be psychic pain and even physical disorders.

Frequently African church leaders have consulted with me about various physical complaints. During the examination, I often find a string tied around the waist to which are attached one or more superstitious charms. While proclaiming faith and trust in God, they are trusting in occult traditional practices of healing. When we have been able to help them resolve these conflicting beliefs, the physical complaints disappear.

I have had personal experience with inner conflicts of values. When I was a single student in medical school, I developed a relationship with an attractive young woman on the hospital staff. As the relationship grew, I became increasingly aware that we had serious conflicts in beliefs and values. I was already preparing for medical mission service and knew in my heart that Ginny would not fit into this type of service or lifestyle. Yet my heart was pulling me strongly toward her. I experienced chest pains that prompted a visit to the medical school infirmary. After extensive tests, including X-rays and an electrocardiogram, I was given the diagnosis of "medical student disease." This, translated, meant inner stress.

One lovely spring afternoon I sat on the bank of the Genesee River and talked to God. In prayer I gave up my relationship to Ginny and told God that, unless he gave a clear indication otherwise, I would not see her again. Three results occurred almost immediately. I felt immense relief (permanently). I felt lonely (temporarily). And the pain disappeared. Inner conflicts of beliefs can have serious consequences.

Of the Ten Commandments, the first commandment—"Worship no god but me" (Exodus 20:3)—is the most important one for our psychological and physical health. Jesus reiterated the significance of this instruction when he gave us the Great Commandment, "Love the Lord your God with all your heart, with all your soul, and with all your mind" (Matthew 22:37).

Putting It All Together

Medical science searches for physical causes of diseases—bacteria, viruses, some sort of parasite, a nutritional or chemical imbalance, or a toxic substance. Health professionals and medical technology have many ways to search for and deal with these possible causes.

Psychology has broadened the search for causes by showing how worry, stress, broken relationships, and painful emotions can cause illness. These factors also require treatment.

If we are to understand and benefit from the spiritual factor of faith in God as part of the healing process, we must understand the role of spiritual causes in the development and progress of illness. Sin is rebellion; it distorts relationships and has serious repercussions on our health and on our response to illness. The forgiveness of sin and the healing of the effects of sin greatly facilitate the healing of many illnesses and diseases.

For adequate healing to take place, the many factors involved in a particular illness—physical, social, emotional, and spiritual—need to be addressed effectively and in concert.

Disorder has come into the social, psychological, and spiritual realms as well as into the physical world. We are responsible in part for this disorder because of our sin. We have broken many relationships, and the resulting alienation opens the door to many kinds of disease. The good news is that there is hope, there is a remedy. Sin is a problem of the heart. God has provided a solution for sin and for our heart problems. We will turn to this now.

7

What's Jesus Got to Do with It?

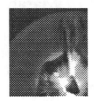

The Old Testament says that by the wounds of Christ we are healed.[1] The New Testament affirms that.[2] For many years I interpreted this "spiritually": I presumed it meant that Jesus could heal the spirit. He gives us salvation, eternal life, and a place in heaven. Because I had been brought up in the Western mindset, which divides the spirit from the body, I couldn't see Christ's healing going beyond the spirit. Healing the body was up to medical science.

Christ does indeed give us salvation, and the Bible makes it clear that salvation is a process. It begins at the new birth when a person makes a commitment to Jesus Christ. Salvation should then progress throughout life as the person grows in spiritual maturity. It becomes complete only in eternity.

In the same way, healing is a journey. It will always be incomplete in this life. Full healing will come only when, after the death of our physical body, we enter into the presence of God in eternity.

The important practical question we will consider now is how faith in Christ can facilitate the healing of particular illnesses as we move forward in our earthly journey. Jesus came to heal the brokenhearted and to bind up their wounds (Psalm 147:3). We have already seen how this can help the healing of many physical diseases. How can Jesus heal our hearts? Why do our hearts need healing?

The Bitter Water of Marah

Back in the book of Exodus is a tiny story of immense significance. It is a symbolic account of God's solution to the problems of our hearts caused by sin. I consider it one of the most meaningful stories in the Bible, for it explains our need for radical healing. It is an Old Testament illustration of a New Testament truth, a symbolic account of how Christ heals us. We find the story in Exodus 15:22-26:

> Then Moses led the people of Israel away from the Red Sea into the desert of Shur. For three days they walked through the desert, but found no water. Then they came to a place called Marah, but the water there was so bitter that they could not drink it. That is why it was named Marah (bitter). The people complained to Moses and asked, "What are we going to drink?" Moses prayed earnestly to the Lord, and the Lord showed him a piece of wood, which he threw into the water; and the water became fit to drink.
>
> There the Lord gave them laws to live by, and there he also tested them. He said, "If you will obey me completely by doing what I

consider right and by keeping my commands, I will not punish you with any of the
diseases that I brought on the Egyptians. I
am the Lord, the one who heals you."

The children of Israel had spent more than four hundred years as slaves in the land of Egypt. Now, by
God's power and mighty intervention, they had
crossed the Red Sea. God had delivered them from
bondage to the Egyptians, and they were now on their
way to the land of liberty and promise. After much rejoicing, Moses gave the order for them to start the
long journey to the Promised Land.

One can picture the mothers and fathers filling up
every available gourd, clay pot, and wineskin with
drinking water, knowing they were to proceed into
arid desert country. They had no Rand-McNally road
atlas to follow, nor could they count on rest stops
along the way. On the first day, when the children
complained of thirst, there was water to drink. On the
second day, the parents cautioned them to drink only
a little, because no one knew when they would find
more water. On the third day, the supplies of water
were gone, the children were crying of thirst, and
anxiety began to mount.

Suddenly someone in the lead shouted "Water!"
and began running toward a spring in the distance.
Others followed in hot pursuit, and they fell to their
knees on the ground beside the spring and scooped
up handfuls of water. But instantly they spit it out on
the ground. The water was so bitter that no one could
drink it.

In utter frustration they turned on Moses. Moses,
wise man that he was, took the problem to the Lord.
The Lord said, "No problem. Look over there. You
see that dead tree? Drag it over to the spring and

throw it into the water." All eyes were on Moses as he lifted this heavy, dead tree trunk and threw it into the water. Undoubtedly many wondered what the old man was doing. Their wonder turned to amazement as the log slowly descended out of sight into the depths of the spring, the water around it gurgling. After a few minutes, Moses took the first sip. When he pronounced the water sweet, they all drank to their fill.

Notice verse 26, which says that it was here that God gave Israel laws to live by and here that he tested them. He laid down a fundamental principle of life: Obedience to him and to his laws leads to life and peace. Disobedience, however, leads to the multitude of problems from which the people of the world (in their case, the Egyptians) suffer.

We need to understand that the Hebrew people interpreted evil events such as diseases as God's punishment for their sins. Moses quotes God as saying that he would punish the people of Israel with diseases if they did not obey his laws, just as he had punished the Egyptians with diseases.

In this day and culture, we tend to look for secondary causes of bad events. We interpret God's statement in this story to mean that when we disobey the laws of God, diseases of one kind or another may come as the result of our disobedience. This puts the responsibility back on us. When we disobey God's laws, we suffer, because that is the way God has made the world.

Bitterness in Our Hearts

What does this story mean? What is the relation between this spring of bitter water, the log, God giving laws to his people, and God being our healer?

The history of the children of Israel is actual history. This episode at Marah took place as it is recorded. However, the history of Israel is more than just any history. It is an allegory of the spiritual history of each one of us. In chapter 2 we talked about the importance of symbols and how our hearts interpret and understand symbols. The stories of the Old Testament are more than just historical accounts. They are stories with meaning; they are symbols for our lives. They symbolize our own spiritual journey through life, pointing out valuable lessons we need to learn for our own growth and maturity. Paul explained this principle to the Christians in Corinth: "All of these things happened to them (Israel) as examples for others, and they were written down as a warning for us" (1 Corinthians 10:11).

Israel spent centuries in bondage to the Egyptians, and she could not save herself. This represents our own bondage to sin and that we cannot save ourselves by our own power. God, by his mighty power, saved Israel from her bondage in Egypt by leading her through the Red Sea. God, by his mighty power acting through Christ, has saved all who trust in him from bondage to sin. The crossing of the Red Sea symbolizes our salvation by God's mighty power and is reason for great rejoicing. Israel quickly discovered, however, that being saved from slavery in Egypt did not solve all her problems. Among the many problems now to be faced was that of clean water to drink; the only available water was too bitter. What is the bitter water's spiritual significance for Israel and for us?

In the Bible, in world literature, in most mythologies, and even in the language of dreams, water symbolizes spirit. This story from Exodus about bitter water has important meaning for us. Salvation frees us from bondage to sin, but it does not purify our spirits. The bitterness of envy, jealousy, anger, and unresolved conflicts and tensions of our hearts is still there. Although we have been saved from sin by the power of God through Christ, our hearts remain polluted with negative emotions that continue to affect our life and influence our health. What is the solution?

David Seamands, Methodist pastor and counselor, writes, "We preachers have often given people the mistaken idea that the new birth and being 'filled with the Spirit' are going to automatically take care of these emotional hang-ups. But this just isn't true. A great crisis experience of Jesus Christ, as important and eternally valuable as this is, is not a shortcut to emotional health. It is not a quickie cure for personality problems."[3]

Israel had been saved from slavery in Egypt by God's power as he brought them across the Red Sea. The people of Israel could not purify the water of Marah, but God provided the solution for their problem. That solution was in a piece of wood which, when thrown into the spring, purified the water. In the same way, God has saved us from slavery to sin through our faith in Jesus Christ, but our emotions, memories, and desires are still polluted by evil. We cannot purify our own hearts of the bitterness of envy, guilt, fear, anger, pride, selfishness, lust, jealousy, or any other "pollutants." As with Israel, God has provided a solution for us. And I don't think it is a coincidence that the water of Marah was purified by a piece of wood—and Christ purified us by his death on a cross of wood.

In the Exodus story, God did not purify the water of Marah. However, he provided the solution and told Moses how to apply it. Fortunately for the people of Israel, Moses did apply it and the people drank pure water. Likewise, God says that the blood of Jesus Christ can purify our conscience from dead works to serve the living God (Hebrews 9:14). It is available, but we must apply it to our minds and hearts in order to become pure.

Have you ever wondered why so many of us Christians have bad tempers, fly off the handle, or become obsessed with material things? In spite of salvation and the assurance of eternal life, many of us live in fear, insecurity, bitterness, or anger, and this makes us difficult to live with or to work with in constructive relationships. We have "crossed the Red Sea," but have not applied the cross or Christ's purifying blood to our inner lives. You may have nagging inner problems, even psychic pain, which you cannot remove from your heart.

One day some years ago Mr. Kihani, the chauffeur of our hospital pick-up truck, returned from a trip on which he'd taken supplies to several of our rural health centers. While he was going up a hill, he saw an elderly woman struggling along the road, carrying a heavy basket of cassava roots on her head with a stack of firewood on top of that. He stopped and helped her get into the back of the truck so he could take her to her village. When he started up, he glanced in the rearview mirror and saw her sitting there with the heavy basket back up on top of her head. He stopped and told her to put the basket on the floor of the truck; he had put her into the truck so that she wouldn't have to carry it. She refused and kept the load on her head all the way to her village. Mr. Kihani laughed heartily each time he told this story to our staff.

The story has a deeper meaning. Many of us carry heavy burdens that Christ longs to take from us. Grudges, bitterness, resentments, anger, even hatred fill our hearts. We refuse to forgive someone who has wronged us, and we suffer from the resulting pent-up, destructive emotions. Did Christ die in vain? So it would seem, at least as far as our healing is concerned. From these burdens can come high blood pressure, stomach disorders, painful arthritis, and troubled breathing.

Salvation and Purification Are Different

When I came to believe in Jesus and committed my life to him, I was saved from the eternal consequences of my sin. I had, in a symbolic way, been led through the waters of the Red Sea by God's power.

I discovered, however, that I still became angry. I continued to succumb to temptations. Fear, jealousy, and envy still occupied rooms in my heart, and my selfish ambition remained. Feelings of rejection, alienation, and shame continued to influence my thoughts and behavior, and even my health. The Spirit of Christ lived in me, but so also did these bitter feelings. Because of this, my life as a Christian was inconsistent, and on many occasions I became miserable because I was torn up inside. Sometimes I would even have chest pain because of this. I would get into conflicts with my family members, my friends, or my associates, or I would withdraw in silent anger. The bitterness of unresolved heart problems not only kept me in inner pain, but it also poisoned my relationships with God and with others. Often it would lead me to say or do things that brought shame to the name of Christ. I was like the woman in the back of Mr. Kihani's pick-up, accepting the invitation to be carried, but continuing to balance a heavy load on my head.

We must recognize, therefore, that salvation is not identical with the purification of the heart, or "sanctification" as it has been called. Salvation is the beginning of a new life and journey. But in the course of this journey there must be ongoing cleansing of our lives, because bitterness in its many forms creeps into us every day. Only the blood of Christ can purify our hearts.

This brings us to a key question, one that has caused dissension and division in the church for centuries. Why did God choose blood as a symbol for healing?

Why the Blood?

The Bible says, "The life of every living being is in the blood" (Leviticus 17:11). Our biomedical sciences have amply demonstrated the truth of this word from the Old Testament. The cells of our entire body depend on the blood for their functioning. Blood transports oxygen and food to every cell and removes the waste products that accumulate in them. It is essential for regulating the temperature, acidity, and mineral balance throughout the body. The hormones that control growth and the activity of many organs are carried to every part of the body by the blood. Blood is our principal line of defense against infection. The white blood cells destroy many invading organisms and produce antibodies against many disease-producing bacteria and viruses. Our whole system of immunity depends on the viability of all elements of our blood. It is our blood, therefore, which sustains life, nourishes us, purifies our system of toxic wastes, regulates our internal environment and activities, and protects us from many diseases. Our life is indeed in the blood.

Day and night, year after year, blood perfuses the whole body and nourishes our organs, tissues, and cells. If the flow of blood to the brain is interrupted for as much as four minutes, brain cells begin to die.

Other organs or members of the body die when deprived of blood. Blood is the vital fluid of our life.

On many occasions I have performed an emergency operation on someone in whom the blood supply to part of the intestines has been cut off by a disease process. It may be a strangulated hernia, or a loop of bowel twisted on itself. The first task is to remove the cause of the constricted circulation so the blood can return to that segment of the bowel. I then simply stand for a few minutes and watch. If I see the blood vessels begin to pulsate, a pink blush replace the bluish-black color of the bowel, and tiny movements begin in the muscles of the intestinal wall, I know that life will return. On the other hand, if I see none of these signs, then I know that the blood supply has been interrupted for too long. That segment of the bowel is now dead and I must remove it.

Blood symbolizes life. Our hearts know this, and in the Bible, in world literature, even in dreams, blood signifies life. By the same token, the losing of blood signifies death. As blood flows from the body, life flows out as well. Blood is therefore one of the most powerful symbols of our spirit.

Blood Sacrifices

In many cultures, including the Hebrew culture, blood sacrifices are used as symbols both of the forgiveness of sin and of the healing of many illnesses. An animal is sacrificed, and its blood is sprinkled on the sinner or on the person who is or has been sick. This speaks to the heart: "You are forgiven," or "You are healed. The life of another being has been shed to heal you of sin and its consequences." When the sinner or the sick person understands the real meaning of the sacrifice, the guilt of sin or the fear, anxiety, and shame of the illness can be healed. The heart understands, "Another died for me. I am now alive and healed."

However, animal sacrifices are cheap. Whenever someone commits a gross sin and feels guilty about it, it is easy to take a goat, a chicken, or a pigeon and kill it as a sacrifice. The gravity of sin is diminished, for forgiveness is now worth only the price of a goat or a bird. The heart knows that. It recognizes that sin has not been dealt with adequately, nor have the wounds and scars of sin been truly healed. For this reason, people made sacrifices over and over again to try to pay the price of sin. But it was never sufficient, for sin is very costly.

Something more is required. What is required for the complete healing of heart, mind, and spirit of the fear, guilt, and shame of sin is the *life blood of God himself*, the God-who-became-man, Jesus Christ, the Anointed One, the Messiah. So this is what God did, and why he did it. Jesus shed his own blood and died to provide adequate healing of the sin in our hearts and to restore us to life.

The next question is how the shedding of Christ's blood makes healing available to us.

Jesus in Gethsemane

On the night before his crucifixion, in the grove of olive trees called Gethsemane just outside the city of Jerusalem, Jesus fought the greatest battle in human history. All the forces of evil were gathered there to contend with our Lord—hatred and pride, lust, greed, deceit, jealousy, guilt, shame and envy. The power of evil was so overwhelming that Jesus was in great agony of soul. Luke reports that blood tinged the sweat that poured from his brow as he wrestled with what he had to do.

The powers of evil wanted to put Jesus to flight and to keep him from going to the cross. They almost succeeded. When Jesus realized that he must take all these evil powers into himself, he begged his Father to find some other way. No other way was possible, so after much agony of spirit, Jesus accepted the task before him.

In utter loneliness, Jesus wrestled within his own spirit. He who had known no sin had to take all of these evil powers into his own heart and carry them to the cross where they would kill him. I do not believe that God put the weight of our sins on a passive, resigned Jesus. I am convinced that Jesus, in full awareness of the horror of sin, actively and willingly took our sin into himself. He did this for three reasons:

- to take from us the necessity of dying for our own sins
- to free us from the hold that sin has over our thoughts, feelings, and desires
- to heal the wounds that sin makes in our hearts

He who had never known pride, envy, hatred, murder, or lust, took them into his own heart. During that long, horrible hour Jesus embraced all the evil powers that try to destroy us. With the sin of all the ages staining his whole being, Jesus walked back to Jerusalem, stood on trial for us, was beaten, then struggled up Calvary's hill with the cross on which he died. "Christ himself carried our sins in his body to the cross" (1 Peter 2:24).

At the Cross

The intensity of Jesus' suffering on the cross is beyond our comprehension. The physical suffering of crucifixion itself is frightful, but Jesus suffered in his spirit far more than in his body. On the cross, Jesus had become sin for us, and God, his heavenly Father, could not be present with him or even look on his Son. From the depths of his spirit, Jesus cried in great anguish, "My God, my God, why did you abandon me?" (Matthew 27:46). Our alienation from God became Jesus' own in order to make possible our restoration to God.

Jesus suffered until his human body could endure the stress no longer. He died probably of heart failure and asphyxia, which terminated when his heart muscle ruptured. When he died, our sin died with him. "We all, like sheep, have gone astray, each of us has turned to his own way, but the LORD has laid on him the iniquity of us all" (Isaiah 53:6, NIV).

Victory over Death

"Let us give thanks to the God and Father of our Lord Jesus Christ. Because of his great mercy, he has given us new life by raising Christ from death. This fills us with a living hope" (1 Peter 1:3-4). The power of sin had killed Jesus; it had ruptured the muscles of his heart. But in the tomb his mortal physical body was transformed into an eternal physical body. His heart muscle was restored, his wounds were healed although the scars remained, and he came forth from the tomb with immortal life.

Joseph's garden tomb was empty on the morning of the third day. This is a well-established historical fact. The guards knew it and so did the women and Peter and John. Certainly the Jewish high priest and his colleagues knew it, for more than likely they visited the tomb to confirm it for themselves. Finding the tomb empty, its covering stone lying on the ground, their only recourse was to bribe the guards to tell a false story. The empty tomb stands above all human history to proclaim that death is no longer the end to human life.[4]

The Healing Symbols

The cross, Christ's blood shed for us, and the empty tomb are symbols that have immense power to heal the broken heart and the wounded spirit. They help to heal our alienation from God, the author of life, and to free us from sin and the fear of death in our hearts and in our bodies.

The cross
The Roman cross was a cruel instrument of death. Jesus, by voluntarily dying on it for us, transformed it into a symbol of life and of love. When I remember the evil things I have done and their consequences on my life and often on the lives of others, I tremble with fear and agony of spirit. But when I realize that Jesus, because he loved me, took the sin and evil of my life into his own heart and died for it on the cross in my place, I come face to face with his amazing love. And that love heals my broken heart and restores my spirit.

Jesus' shed blood
Jesus' blood gave life to his physical body when he was the God-man in our midst. He voluntarily gave his blood on the cross to restore life to our hearts. When we accept the symbol of Jesus' blood—the blood of the Lamb of God—and apply it to our thoughts, emotions, and desires, his blood can heal our hearts of the pain that sin has caused. This healing brings the inner peace that strengthens our bodies.

The empty tomb

The empty tomb is the symbol that heals us of the fear of death. It is the sign of the transformation that awaits all who come to Christ—the transformation of our souls from this limited, marred environment to the free, eternal environment in God's presence. The empty tomb says that death, our greatest enemy, was overcome when Christ rose from the dead. Jesus' resurrection overcame the power of the destructive thoughts, emotions, and desires that weaken the immune system and cause disorder in many of our physical organs. Although physical death will eventually come to all of us, the tomb symbolizes the transformation of our earthly physical bodies into the immortal physical bodies that will endure forever. The empty tomb is our living hope, and this hope brings healing.

The Healing Power of Christ's Presence in the Heart

In addition to bringing us the healing power of these symbols, Jesus heals in a second way. He heals by his own presence in our hearts.

When a person invites Christ to come into his or her life—heart—where does he go? Where does he stay? Let us look again at the symbol of the heart as a home with many rooms and see into which rooms Christ comes and where he stays. Even though this is a somewhat artificial picture, it is nevertheless highly instructive because it enables our hearts to intuit and thus understand better where Jesus lives within us.

Inviting Christ into the heart is a conscious decision, and the Spirit of Jesus enters into the conscious mind. This experience has an effect on our feelings and emotions. However, Jesus is a gentleman. He will not enter into any of the "rooms" of the subconscious mind unless he is invited. Jesus will not disturb, change, or heal our beliefs, emotions, feelings, or desires unless we ask him to do so.

I was converted, or "saved," when I consciously invited Jesus to come into my life. Jesus came in, and my spirit became alive. However, I allowed Jesus to come into only a small part of my life. I gave him access only to a limited area of my personality. I had stuff down there I could not deal with and was too ashamed of to present to Jesus. In other areas, I had been hurt so badly that I shut them off even to myself.

I eventually learned that it is these sealed-off parts of the heart that exert a strong influence over our psychological and even physical health. It is in these parts of the personality where Christ's healing presence is so important. Here is where a competent Christ-centered counselor can give invaluable help in enabling us to open more areas of the heart to the healing power of the presence of Jesus Christ.

This raises an important question. Does becoming a Christian help the healing process? From the medical, psychological, and spiritual standpoints, the answer is yes. Is it necessary to become a Christian in order to be healed? Not necessarily, because God has provided to everyone many different means to health and healing—right in our bodies, and in medical science. Coming into a personal relationship with Jesus Christ promotes health and healing, but a person can indeed get well without encountering Jesus. I can list, however, at least three ways in which a personal relationship with Jesus Christ can promote healing.

1. A *relationship with Jesus gives new meaning to life.* When a person chooses to be committed to Christ, life takes on a new meaning. He or she now has a place to be somebody, a place of value in earthly history and in eternity. Knowing that one is a child of God gives dignity to life and a sense of eternal value. Being affirmed by God is quickly translated into self-affirmation and the inner assurance of being in God's family. God said to his people Israel, "Do not be afraid—I will save you. I have called you by name— you are mine" (Isaiah 43:1).

This deep assurance gives to the heart the peace that promotes healing and strengthens health. This is what happened to the woman with bleeding whose case history we studied in chapter 2. The word of assurance from Jesus—when her heart accepted it— healed the woman's spirit, soul, and body.

2. A relationship with Jesus provides a reason to live.

When I became a Christian, I had a reason to live beyond my own interests. My life took on purpose. When we have something to live for, the physical self responds positively.

Nellie's husband was the principal of our high school in Africa. He died in our hospital in 1985 after more than a year of unsuccessful treatment of many strange infections. Shortly before he died, the serological test for AIDS became available, and we found that both he and his wife were sero-positive. They had already lost two small babies to repeated infections that were probably from AIDS. Nellie was now left with three sero-negative, school-aged children to raise. In her intense grief, Nellie's spirit almost broke, and her already affected immune system was seriously compromised by the end of 1985.

Some of our Christian mothers took Nellie into their care. They shared their own meager resources with her. Most of all, they shared Jesus with her, and Nellie opened her heart to Christ. Joy came into her life, her repeated infections cleared up, and she went into remission. She determined in her heart to live long enough to see her three children come into the kingdom of Christ and the oldest two finish high school. She also wanted to use every opportunity to tell the truth about AIDS to other young people. Because of the extreme poverty of our people in Congo, we can offer them none of the expensive anti-HIV medications available in North America and Europe. Whenever Nellie got an infection, she had no medical treatment other than antibiotics.

Nellie and my wife, Miriam, became like sisters. One day Nellie's anger spilled over and she exclaimed, "Why did my husband do this to me? Why did he give me this fatal infection and then abandon me?" Before Miriam could say a word, Nellie's spirit softened, and with a radiant smile she said, "But if I had not gotten AIDS, I would never have come to know Jesus."

Nellie's three children came to know Jesus in a real way. The oldest two had graduated from high school by 1994. Nellie then told Miriam she was ready to go home. In May of 1995, ten years after her diagnosis of HIV disease, Nellie entered joyfully into the presence of Jesus. Her immune system had wrestled against this infection and had coped with the virus for almost ten years because Jesus lived in her heart and had given her reasons to live.

3. A relationship with Jesus brings freedom from fear.

All of us deal with fear—fear of death, cancer, abandonment, poverty, violence, and so forth. Fear is a powerful emotion that can inhibit the immune system and slow down healing.

Faith in Jesus Christ is more than just an intellectual exercise or a psychological condition. When Jesus comes into the heart of a person, *he is really there*. Jesus is a powerful presence and a protective shield. When Mrs. Matala explained this to John, the young man with tuberculosis whom we discussed in chapter 1, his fear was healed. He recognized that an invisible yet solid wall of love surrounded him, which the malevolent power of his uncle's curse could not penetrate. When John's heart accepted that as reality, his white blood cells became more effective and he began to recover.

With Christ living in our hearts, we have the assurance of his protection. No matter what the circumstances, I know that Christ is present within me to help me. I can thus live in confidence and sleep in peace. This is the peace of mind that makes the body strong.

8

Heart Cleaning

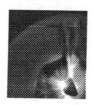

The term "spring cleaning" brings back fond memories for me. I can still see a Baptist parsonage, already a hundred years old, in a small town in upstate New York. The warm spring air is circulating through windows opened for the first time in six months. Rugs are draped across clotheslines in the yard, waiting for my small arms to wield the rugbeater and whack the dust from them. Mattresses have been laid out on the grass to air, while Mother carefully cleans the dust from the bedsprings, and I am charged with sweeping the layers of accumulated pillow feathers from underneath them. Spring-cleaning was a tradition, and the welcome smell of freshness that permeated the house afterwards made the tedious efforts worthwhile.

In chapter 5, I likened the heart to a home—one having many rooms in which much is stored away. So much dust, debris, and garbage can accumulate in those rooms! What can be done to clean our inner house of its accumulated rubbish? Is it possible for the heart to be cleaned just as the old parsonage was cleaned?

Heart Sickness

Jeremiah wrote, "Who can understand the human heart? There is nothing else so deceitful; it is too sick to be healed" (Jeremiah 17:9). We have seen how difficult it is to understand ourselves. With all that is buried in our memories, we can't possibly be aware of all that is in our heart. The root of sinful deceit goes so deep into our thoughts and imaginations that we are blind to our own condition. Self-deception makes true self-knowledge impossible.

Jeremiah then calls on the Lord for healing, saying, "Heal me, O Lord, and I will be healed" (17:14). He believed that although no person could heal him, God could. The heart can never be completely healed in this life. Sin and disorder are too deeply imbedded in the psyche of all of us. The good news is that much *can* be healed. Our hearts can be healed by Jesus' presence and by the power of his blood.

In this chapter we will not discuss the full range of methods for "heart cleaning." Psychology, psychiatry, and the various forms of counseling have numerous approaches to our heart struggles. A person with heart problems can benefit from any or all of these methods.

Unfortunately, religion and science have been at odds with each other for at least as long as there's been such a science as psychiatry. The scientific disciplines and the faith traditions have not sought to understand one another; they have spent more energy finding fault with each other.

Many expressions of the Christian faith have indeed wandered into error and engaged in practices contrary to the Word of Christ. This does not, however, invalidate the fundamental proclamation of the Christian faith that Jesus is the Way, the Truth, and the Life. Our incomplete and often erroneous understanding of spiritual healing does not negate Jesus as our healer.

Psychology has likewise strayed into error, on occasion proclaiming and practicing incomplete, erroneous, or even harmful methods. Nevertheless, we are psychological beings, and it is essential that we continue our scientific study of the psyche.

This unnecessary antagonism between necessary disciplines is tragic. Each one is promoting an incomplete yet important understanding of who we are as persons. Psychology on its own, and spiritual healing on its own, are insufficient.[1]

Science and faith are in fact complementary. But for Christians the Bible is the final authority. The Bible is God's Word; in it God has revealed the truth about himself, about us as persons, and about our many relationships. The Bible also speaks about sin, its consequences, and the remedies God has provided. Healing involves restoration of relationships and restoration of souls and bodies that have been damaged by sin, sickness, or both.

We can embrace wholeheartedly any psychological technique that helps us restore our relationships in the way God intends. Any technique based on an understanding of human life not supported by God's Word, however scientific it may purport to be, can be harmful.[2]

The presence of Christ in the heart can often penetrate to the very center of a heart problem and heal it. Added to biblically sound methods of psychology, psychiatry, and pastoral counseling, Christ-centered counseling can reach the depths of the soul and spirit, healing and integrating them, and allowing the healed heart to strengthen the body.

Healing and Fear

Fear is a normal emotional reaction to a situation that seems to pose a threat to us. If dealt with quickly and properly, it rarely causes ill effects to our health. However, if we do not deal with the fear properly but hold onto it, it can become harmful. Fear can affect the muscle tone of our arteries, bronchial tubes, or intestinal tract; it can cause diverse pains, including chronic headache, and a multitude of other symptoms. On many occasions we bury the cause of our fear in our memory so that identification and resolution become difficult.

Mrs. Kilenda is the wife of a dynamic pastor in a large city in the Congo. This pastor has worked hard to mobilize churches in the fight against AIDS. Their marriage has been stable, and they have seven healthy children, some of whom are now adults. Mrs. Kilenda came to the Vanga Hospital complaining of diffuse pains in her abdomen and back, chronic fatigue, and difficulty sleeping. These symptoms had bothered her for two years.

I could find no physical signs of illness, so I presumed she was suffering from psychological distress of some sort. I referred her to Mrs. Matala for further questioning and counseling.

Mrs. Matala spent several hours with Mrs. Kilenda, and referred her back to me frequently. Neither Mrs. Matala nor I could identify the cause of this woman's symptoms, but she kept telling me, "Doctor, I hurt." On the fourth visit, in some frustration, I almost made the mistake that we physicians should never make but often do, telling such a person, "I can't find anything wrong with you," or "It's all in your head," or, even worse, "You are not sick." The latter would be 100 percent wrong because she was sick and she knew it.

So I explained that up to this point we had not found the cause of her symptoms. We had done almost all possible examinations. The only other examination we could do was to test her for AIDS, which I thought was quite unnecessary. However, she said, "Doctor, please test me for whatever you can." So she went to the lab for an HIV test.

Three days later she returned to me for the results. When I told her that her AIDS test was negative, she immediately leaned forward and demanded, "Are you sure?"

"Absolutely. Our AIDS test is practically 100 percent reliable."

To my astonishment, she sat back in her chair and heaved a big sigh. She was healed! It was now my turn to lean forward and ask her, "Mrs. Kilenda, you mean to say you have been afraid you had AIDS?"

She began to weep as she told me that two years previously she had had a severe attack of malaria. Her husband took her to the hospital, where they gave her an intravenous infusion. As she watched the staff put the needle into her arm, she was sure it was contaminated with the AIDS virus. So she had lived and suffered with this fear—fear that had caused all of her symptoms—but had been too ashamed to tell anyone about it. The healing word that her heart had longed to hear had just been pronounced: "Your AIDS test is negative." The following day she returned to Kikwit to rejoin her family, feeling just fine.

Healing and Guilt

The feeling of guilt is a sense of having done wrong and a sense that the wrong is known by another person or by God. The offense may be real or imagined; in either event, the sorrow is very real and painful.

The profound feelings of remorse can cause much emotional distress and can even lead to physical illness.

David Belgum believes that up to 75 percent of people in hospitals with physical illnesses have sicknesses rooted in emotional causes. These patients are punishing themselves with their illness, Dr. Belgum says. Their physical symptoms and breakdowns may be their involuntary confessions of guilt.[3]

The Genesis account of the Fall (Genesis 3) makes abundantly clear the seriousness of guilt and its consequences. Adam and Eve fled from the presence of God because they knew they had exposed themselves. They were naked spiritually, psychologically, and morally as well as physically. No quantity of fig leaves could cover their exposure or their sense of guilt. However, Christ can heal the remorse of guilt because he can forgive our offenses and our sin.

The word needed to heal the remorse of guilt is the assurance of forgiveness. Both the Old and the New Testaments give us many assurances that God forgives all who confess their sins to him and turn from their sins.

Is restitution also necessary if we are to be healed of our guilt? Usually it is, if it is possible to restore what our sin has harmed. Zaccheus promised restitution of all he had taken illegally (Luke 19:1-10). This was part of his salvation and the healing of his guilt. Where actual restitution is not possible, a commitment to the service of others can become a symbolic means of restitution.

Healing and Bitterness

One day Peter asked Jesus how many times he should forgive someone who kept wronging him. Jesus replied that there was no limit; we should always forgive others. He then told a sobering parable that has much to do with illness.

[Once there was] a king who decided to check on his servants' account. He had just begun to do so when one of them was brought in who owed him millions of dollars. The servant did not have enough to pay his debt, so the king ordered him to be sold as a slave, with his wife and his children and all that he had, in order to pay the debt. The servant fell on his knees before the king, "Be patient with me," he begged, "and I will pay you everything." The king felt sorry for him, so he forgave him the debt and let him go.

Then the man went out and met one of his fellow servants who owed him a few dollars. He grabbed him and started choking him. "Pay back what you owe me!" he said. His fellow servant fell down and begged him, "Be patient with me, and I will pay you back." But he refused; instead, he had him thrown into jail until he should pay the debt. When the other servants saw what happened, they were very upset and went to the king and told him everything. So he called the servant in. "You worthless slave!" he said. "I forgave you the whole amount you owed me, just because you asked me to. You should have had mercy on your fellow servant, just as I had mercy on you." The king was very angry, and he sent the servant to jail to be punished until he should pay back the whole amount.

And Jesus concluded, "That is how my Father in heaven will treat every one of you unless you forgive your brother from your heart." (Matthew 18:23-35)

Each one of us owes God an immense debt because of our sin and disobedience. We cannot repay such a debt, but God through Christ has paid it. When we confess our sins and commit ourselves to following Christ, we are set free from that insurmountable debt.

We all wrong each other. Many times others have wronged us. Jesus is telling us that just as God has forgiven us, we must forgive others. If we do not, there will be consequences. Jesus' final statement is a frightful one and a severe warning for us all: "That is how my Father in heaven will treat every one of you unless you forgive your brother from your heart." God takes our relationships very seriously. He expects us to keep all of our relationships in order. That requires forgiving others when they wrong us.

What will God do to us if we do not forgive someone? What is the "prison" into which he puts us? This does not have to do with our salvation or with hell. Our salvation depends on our faith in what Christ has done for us and not on anything we do ourselves. If our salvation had to do with forgiving every wrong done to us, I doubt any of us would make it!

I believe that the prison Jesus is referring to is the prison of illness. Day after day people come to me with hurts here, pains there, weakness, trouble with their breathing, chronic fatigue, or any number of physical problems. But as we work through the whole history of a person, we often find no physical pathology. What we do find are broken relationships, grudges, and bitterness toward others. When these relational problems are healed, the physical symptoms are often resolved.

Mr. Lisala, a high school principal, came to our hospital some years ago. He was losing weight rapidly because of chronic vomiting and diarrhea. Aside from the weight loss, we could find no signs of illness. Again Mrs. Matala became the healer. As she went through the history, she asked Mr. Lisala if there were any persons with whom he worked who gave him problems. He immediately became very defensive, so Mrs. Matala quickly backed off, knowing she was coming close to this man's real problem. Slowly she worked her way back to interpersonal relationships.

Suddenly Mr. Lisala began spilling out vitriolic hatred toward the school superintendent and the pastor who were responsible for this particular school. According to Mr. Lisala, these were evil men. They were constantly insulting him and doing horrible things to destroy his reputation. As he recounted this, he suddenly vomited all over Mrs. Matala.

Knowing that Mr. Lisala was in no condition to proceed further with the consultation (nor was she!), Mrs. Matala sent him back to his room. The following day, she began asking him what he knew about Christ. He was resistant to Jesus because of the lives of the "Christian" superintendent and pastor. Nevertheless, Mrs. Matala was able to talk to him about Jesus as he really is, and finally Mr. Lisala realized that he needed Christ in his own life. When he accepted Christ, Mrs. Matala knew she could help him deal with his problem.

She read to him many things Christ said about our relationships with others. She also read him the parable in Matthew 18 and talked about the necessity to forgive others the wrongs they have done to us. Mr. Lisala then said an interesting thing: "These men are not my real problem. My problem is in my own reaction to them. Yes, I can forgive them, for now I see they are not bad men." Christ had already changed this man's heart.

After a time of prayer, Mrs. Matala asked him, "Can you now forgive yourself for the reactions you have had to these men?" His heart understood her question, and he readily assented. He confessed to the Lord the anger and resentment he had felt toward these men. He asked the Lord to cleanse him of these destructive emotions and to give him a love for these men. Within a week, Mr. Lisala had regained ten pounds and returned to his home and his work, healed.

What does forgiveness mean? Does it mean to condone what has been done or the person who has done it? By no means. Forgiveness does not diminish the gravity of the sin committed or the evil done. Forgiveness simply means releasing the offending person or persons to Jesus and refusing to condemn them any longer. I no longer condemn in my spirit those who have wronged me. I simply put them in the hands of Christ to work with them as he sees fit and as he is able. Then *I* am set free. But if I do not forgive, I am the one who suffers. I am the one who gets sick. My refusal to forgive does not make the offending person ill; he or she may be totally unaware of my feelings. But it makes me ill, and I need to be healed of this bitterness.

Divorce is one of the most illness-producing events in human life. Millions suffer from the pain of bitterness and the inability to forgive the one who has hurt them. Turning the offending spouse over to Jesus and *leaving him or her there* can be immensely liberating and healing.

Does one have to wait until the other person asks for forgiveness? Absolutely not. If the other person does ask for it, then a reconciliation is possible. Many times, however, the offending person has no intention of asking for forgiveness. He may be far away—or he may even have died years ago. Nevertheless, in prayer I can come to Christ and tell him that I am turning this person over to his love and mercy. I let go of my condemning spirit by releasing that person into the care and judgment of Christ. Then Christ can do his work of healing in my own heart.[4]

Healing and Anger

Paul said to the Ephesians, "When you become angry, do not let your anger lead you into sin, and do not stay angry all day. Don't give the Devil a chance" (Ephesians 4:26-27). There is an amazing amount of psychological truth packed into these two verses.

Anger is a normal human phenomenon; it is an intense emotional response to something that has hurt us or to something we see as hurting someone else. Anger as such is not sinful. Jesus became angry and acted on several occasions on the energy of his anger. He acted to do good things.

The moral aspect of anger is in how we handle it, not in the anger itself. Anger is a surge of intense emotional energy. Either we make decisions about how to direct it, or we allow the emotional energy to lead us into saying or doing things that may be destructive and sinful. Jesus had his anger under perfect control when he cleansed the temple and when he scolded the religious leaders. I believe Jesus even got angry when he saw certain diseases like leprosy and the way they destroyed people.

We don't see Jesus responding with anger when he himself was attacked, insulted, or threatened. His ability to maintain his composure was grounded in his own knowledge of who he was and what he was doing.

Jesus was secure in himself and in the presence of his Father with him. This is perhaps the most important antidote to anger—knowing who we are and being comfortable in what we are doing in the presence of God. If the world attacks us, that is the world's problem.

Paul says that we are not to go to bed angry or to let the sun go down on our anger (Ephesians 4:26, NIV). We know that retained anger is deadly for health. Chronic anger increases gastric acidity; it affects the tone of the muscles of our arteries; and it affects the movement of our intestines. It changes our hormones, and this can lead to chronic inflammation in various organs. Chronic anger is bad news for the health. It gives the devil a chance to make us ill.

When my mother died at the good age of one hundred years, my brother and I were left to dispose of her possessions. Among them were special family heirlooms and some valuable antiques. The thorny question of who should get what fell to us. Among my brother, myself, mother's nieces, nephews, and others who were close to her, certain disagreements arose about some of the family belongings.

A few months later, Miriam and I were participating in a women's retreat. The final event was to be a communion service around a big fireplace. The pastor leading the service asked Miriam and me to speak briefly to the women prior to communion.

That morning I received a letter from a cousin who had been offended and hurt because certain belongings of my mother had not been given to him. I misinterpreted his letter as an accusation and became intensely angry. Why could he not understand the pressures we were under, the grief we were dealing with, and that we had tried to do the best we could for everyone? My heart began to seethe. I knew that if

I were to say anything helpful to the women that evening, my heart had to be at peace. Yet I could not rid myself of the anger and find the peace I needed.

Finally I told Miriam to inform the pastor that I just could not make it that evening. She would have to go it alone. Very lovingly, yet firmly, Miriam asked me, "Dan, how can you tell others how Christ can heal the heart if you cannot let him heal your own?" Ouch! I knew what I had to do.

At the beginning of the service the pastor gave each of us a dry stick. He explained that before we partook of the bread and the cup we were to examine our hearts to see what we might be holding onto that was wrong—resentment, anger, jealousy, or some other sinful thought or feeling. The stick was to be a symbol of our sin, and we would each come to the fireplace, throw it in, and then partake of communion. He then nodded to me to share my few words with the women.

After breathing a quick prayer for help, I briefly told the women the story of what had happened regarding mother's belongings. I confessed the anger and bitterness that churned in my heart against my cousin. I held up the stick and said that I was putting the anger and bitterness on that stick of wood. I turned to the fire, threw it in, and watched it burn up. As I did, the anger and bitterness dissipated, and the peace of Jesus replaced them.

That burning stick was the healing symbol my heart needed. It spoke to me because, with Miriam's and God's help, I found the courage before these ladies to confess my sin and need for healing. As a result, my anger was gone before sunset and the devil had to slink away. When I ate the bread and drank of the cup, the assurance of forgiveness and heart cleansing came, and I was set free.

Healing and Memories

Memories of events even from earliest childhood can cause negative emotions to rise, dark feelings to weigh heavily, and hurtful thoughts to torment us inwardly. The good news is that these painful memories can be healed by the power of Christ.

Some years ago my wife and I attended a teaching seminar on healing led by Bishop Cox, who was then the Episcopal Bishop for the Diocese of Oklahoma. Mrs. Cox spoke to us and told a striking story. She said that God had given her a gift of knowledge. Often, as her husband would be speaking or teaching, she would receive a strong inner impression that someone in the audience was suffering from a particular illness or infirmity and that God could heal that person. She would quickly write a note and give it to an usher to take to her husband. At the end of his message, he would then ask the audience if there was someone present with the type of problem his wife had described. In many cases, her impression was correct, and the person with that type of illness would come forward for prayer and be healed.

In one particular healing seminar, she received a strong impression that the healthy-looking young man sitting beside her had a serious breathing problem because he had been born with the umbilical cord wrapped tightly around his neck. She did not know how to handle this revelation, for the young man was a total stranger to her and he seemed perfectly healthy. It so happened he was the organist in the church where the seminar was held. After the seminar, she began discussing music with him and they became acquainted with each other. Finally she felt free to ask him if he suffered from a breathing problem.

When he asked in astonishment how she knew that,

she explained the gift God had given her and the impression she had received that he had difficulty breathing. He told her that since his earliest childhood, he could not sleep flat in bed. If he tried, he would suffocate. He always had to sleep propped up on several pillows. His parents had taken him to many physicians, and he'd had multiple examinations in some leading medical institutions, all revealing no signs of disease. "Yet," he said, "I cannot sleep lying down."

The young man's mother was present. She joined the conversation and confirmed what her son had explained. Mrs. Cox inquired about the pregnancy and the birth, and the mother assured her that all had been normal. When Mrs. Cox asked if the baby had cried immediately at birth, or had he had some difficulty breathing, the mother suddenly recalled that there had been a brief problem. She remembered the doctors rushing around trying to do something with her infant son, because the umbilical cord had been wrapped tightly around his neck and he was not breathing. The baby soon began crying lustily and seemed perfectly normal, so the mother had quickly forgotten the incident. Mrs. Cox's inspired diagnosis was now confirmed.

Mrs. Cox asked the young man if he wanted to be healed. When he readily assented, she called her husband, the bishop, to come and explained the situation to him. After a few questions to the young man, the bishop prayed. In his prayer he simply asked Jesus, whom he knew was in the heart of the young man, to speak a word of healing to the deepest part of his memory. He asked Jesus to assure this man's heart that he had been present at the birth. He had held him as a tiny baby as he descended the birth canal. He knew the tightness of the cord wrapped around the neck and the suffocation it was causing. It was he, Jesus, who had brought out the head in time, who had helped the doctors and nurses do quickly what was necessary, who had protected the brain from damage, and who had saved his life. The bishop asked Christ to take away from the young man's mind the pain of that terrifying experience and now to allow him to sleep peacefully. The young man was healed in that moment, and he has been able to sleep flat in bed ever since then.[5]

What is "miraculous" about the healing of this young man is the inspired word, which God gave to Mrs. Cox. When she acted on that word and the bishop spoke a healing word in prayer, Christ healed the young man's heart and cured his breathing problem.

Memories from the time of our birth are still present in our hearts, even though most of those memories are lost to conscious recall. Perhaps even memories from the prenatal months influence us in later years. But none of them are beyond the power of Christ to reach and to heal.

9

Free to Be Healthy

As human beings, we consider freedom to be of great value. One of life's great ironies, however, is the enormous propensity of the human spirit for slavery. Freedom brings awesome responsibilities with it—decisions to make, consequences to be accountable for. We prefer to submit to the control of something outside ourselves, something that reduces the necessity for making decisions and for accepting responsibility for those decisions. Unfortunately this diminishes our value as human beings and can also damage our health.

The slavery we choose may take the form of compulsive thoughts and behavior patterns. We cannot change these repetitive habits even though we may expend much energy in trying to do so. Other times the slavery may be to outside substances that we take into ourselves and become dependent on.

Compulsive behavior or substance addiction involves

body, mind, and spirit. They are perhaps the clearest example of how care for the whole person is essential if healing is to be effective.

The Nature of Addiction

An addiction is a condition of biochemical dependency. When a person begins taking an addictive substance, this quickly alters the way brain cells produce certain neurochemicals. In a short while, the body and the brain assume they can no longer function without the addictive substance. Tobacco, alcohol, narcotics, and tranquilizers are major addicting substances. Helping a person break away from the use of the addictive substance is often a long and difficult process, which frequently results in failure.

A similar addictive mechanism occurs in certain repetitive behavior patterns. In this case, however, the addictive substance is one of our own neurochemicals. The brain is the source of the neurochemicals produced as a response to emotions and feelings. These chemicals circulate throughout the body and affect all the organs. The neurochemicals produced as a result of intense pleasure are opioids, similar in chemical structure to opium. Not only do they make the body feel good; they also diminish the perceptions of stress and pain. This explains why opium and its derivatives can have a strong attraction for us; the whole body, as well as the mind, enjoys the effect.

The pleasurable sensations, stress reduction, and pain relief of opioids from the brain, or of opium and heroin from outside the body, are short-lived. They last only a few hours. The body then wants more. After two or three doses of opium or heroin, the production of opioids by the brain is suppressed, and the brain and body become dependent on the external drug. Without regular doses of the drug, intense pain and suffering occur, lasting for days. Drug addiction is therefore like slavery. Escape is very difficult and painful, and it is rarely successful unless there is outside help.

Of all the pleasure-giving activities we do, sexual pleasure is the most intense. It stimulates the brain to produce a surge of opioids which bring a deep sense of satisfaction, fulfillment, and relaxation to the whole body. If a particular action stimulates a surge of pleasure-producing neuropeptides, and this is repeated frequently, the person has difficulty breaking the cycle. The body craves the pleasure-producing neuropeptides stimulated by that particular activity, and a strong habit pattern is formed that is hard to change. Certain compulsive patterns of sexual activity are the result of this type of mechanism. A person becomes addicted to his or her own behavior.[1]

There are many accounts that demonstrate that religious conversion, and especially a genuine experience with Jesus Christ, can result in the breaking of certain addictions, often in quite a dramatic fashion. Consider the following story.

Dr. Jacques Katele has been the medical director of the Vanga Hospital in the Congo for several years. He has been a delight to work with; he is a competent physician with a fine personality. For several years, however, neither Miriam nor I knew what was smoldering inside his heart and his family.

Jacques's parents were faithful church members and took him and his siblings regularly to church. During high school, however, Jacques became adept at finding ways to avoid church. During his first year of medical school he fell in love with Honorine, a Christian girl from a tribe that unfortunately was unacceptable to Jacques's parents. They forbade him to see her under any circumstances, and marriage was totally out of the question. Tension built up in Jacques, and he began suffering chronic headaches and loss of concentration. His studies began to suffer. He went to the neuropsychiatric clinic, where the doctor simply prescribed Valium (diazepam). Jacques found that with the help of Valium he could sleep better and cope with his studies. He soon realized, however, he could not study or sleep without it; he was addicted.

Since parental opposition to marriage to Honorine was insurmountable, Jacques and Honorine had a private ceremony. They started having a family. When Jacques finished his studies, he heard that we were looking for young Congolese physicians, and he came to us as a general practice resident. We were impressed with his abilities, and after his residency he became a member of our staff. In the meantime Honorine became a dear friend of Miriam's. She shared with Miriam her concern about Jacques. Not only was he dependent on valium; he was also consuming increasing quantities of alcoholic beverages. Only some time later did we learn that he was likewise spending time with other women.

Jacques made serious efforts to break his addictions to Valium, alcohol, and sexual indiscretions, but he was unable to do so. Some of our Christian staff members who knew of Jacques's problems spent time counseling him and praying for him. On several occasions, he promised to stop drinking and being unfaithful, but within a day or two he would return to these destructive habits. His family began to suffer. I did research into possible treatments for Valium addiction, only to find that there seemed to be no effective therapy.

One evening a few years later, Jacques's two oldest daughters came into his study and announced that they wanted to leave the family to go live with neighbors. Jacques, who loved his family, was shocked and demanded an explanation. They explained that because of his behavior there was no happiness or peace in their family. When he was drunk, he would often shout at their mother and would even beat her. So they wanted to leave. Jacques was very repentant and promised never to drink again. Nevertheless, the next afternoon after work he was again at the local bar with his friends.

On Pentecost Sunday in 1993, Honorine announced to Jacques that she was taking him to church. He excused himself and said he had much to do at the hospital and would worship the Lord there. So Honorine stormed off to church very upset. To her great surprise, a few minutes later Jacques slipped into the seat beside her dressed in his Sunday best.

Mrs. Matala was preaching that morning, and she used Romans 7 as the basis of her message. She described the Apostle Paul's anguish at trying unsuccessfully to change his inner life and his behavior, ending by exclaiming, "What an unhappy man I am! Who will rescue me from this body that is taking me to death?" He then affirms, "Thanks be to God, who does this through our Lord Jesus Christ!" (Romans 7:24-25).

When Mrs. Matala finished her message, she invited anyone to come forward whose life resembled Paul's and who wanted to be set free. Jacques was the first among many who went forward. Numerous knowing glances were exchanged by some of the hospital staff ("There he goes again"). When Mrs. Matala finished praying for all in the group, Jacques turned to the congregation and declared firmly that Christ had come into the depths of his heart and that he was finished with alcohol and immorality. By doing this, he made himself accountable to the whole congregation for his subsequent behavior.

The next morning it was clear that a genuine change had occurred. Jacques, who had always been kindly and pleasant, was now radiant. Time has proved his declaration true, as more than six years of alcohol-free and moral living have followed. His family has prospered because peace has been restored.

But what about the Valium? Two weeks after Jacques's healing, a big convention of the Hospital Christian Fellowship was held in Brazzaville. Our hospital sent a delegation of ten people, which included Jacques and Mrs. Matala. One evening the speaker from West Africa paused in the middle of his message to say, without knowing why, that there was someone in the audience who was addicted to Valium. If that person wanted to be liberated, Christ could set him or her free.

After the message, Jacques went up to the speaker, put his arm around him, and said he was the person on Valium. He asked him to pray with him. The group from Vanga returned to the dormitory where they were staying. The speaker and the Vanga delegation gathered around Jacques, and the speaker asked him if he wanted to be healed. As his response, Jacques handed him his bottle of Valium with fourteen pills inside, and together they flushed them down the toilet. The group then prayed for Jacques's complete deliverance from the heart problems that had enslaved him to Valium for seventeen years. Jacques was set completely free in that moment.

This story, as well as many others that could be told, indicates that the presence of Jesus Christ in the deep mind, along with a decision of the will and an act of faith, can bring about changes in the physiology of the brain and the production of neuropeptides.

The word of healing for Jacques was, "Thanks be to God, who does this through our Lord Jesus Christ!" (Romans 7:24-25). He combined this with a public act of faith. Christ set Jacques free from three difficult addictive processes: immorality, addiction to alcohol, and dependence on Valium. Physically, psychologically, and spiritually he was set free. Christ is our liberator.

The Nature of Sexuality

Sexuality is one of the deepest parts of our personality. We did not depict it in our diagram of the heart because it pervades the entire heart, from thoughts and memories to the basic instincts. It involves the body as well as the mind and the emotions, desires, and memories. It likewise involves the spirit because gender and sexuality are a major part of who we are as individuals.

The account of creation in Genesis states clearly that masculinity and femininity have come from God and therefore are good. The physical aspect of our sexuality involves hormones, neuropeptides, sexual organs, and connections with other organs, all of which have been created and engineered by God.

Psychologically our sexuality involves our needs for affirmation, intimacy, and security. It also involves our desires for pleasure, sexual fulfillment, creativity, and to a variable extent, power over others. On the spiritual level, our sexuality contributes to an understanding of self and of the meaning and purpose of life. My gender and the masculinity and femininity that go with it are very much a part of who I am as an individual. Furthermore, the Bible uses the intimacy of the sexual relationship as an allegory of the intimate relationship God wants to have with us.

Sexual desires generate powerful internal energies, and these can be difficult to control. God has provided us with resources to help us control and direct these energies.

1. *The presence of Christ within us can give us power to control our emotions, feelings, and drives.* This is what set Jacques free from his habitual immoral behavior.

2. *In the Bible, God has outlined his plan for the fulfillment of our sexuality and the patterns of behavior that are healthy and constructive.* God is concerned about our health, and the laws and commandments that he has provided for all aspects of our lives will promote our health and show us how to have right relationships.

3. *The love, security, example, and biblically based education of parents are invaluable.*

4. *Finally, the encouragement of a strong Christian community is of great importance.* In my father's church, two dozen women met regularly to pray for missions and for specific missionaries. They also prayed for me because they knew I was preparing to be a missionary. They wrote to me often to encourage me and assure me of their prayers. This helped me cope with temptations during my adolescent and young adult years, for I did not want to disappoint these faithful women.

The powerful psychic energies related to our sexuality begin influencing us in very early childhood. We can compare them to fire. Fire is necessary for our life and comfort, and it can be creative; it can also be destructive. To be creative, fire must be in the proper place and adequately controlled. If not, it can be harmful and even deadly. A stable marriage is the "fireplace" God has provided for the fulfillment of our sexual desires (Genesis 2:24-25). Heterosexual union in marriage is good and is blessed by God. It is the only safe and healthy place for sexual union.

Sexuality is part of our personality. God has made us to have sexual desires. The moral aspect of our sexuality lies in how we handle the energies that our sexual desires stir up within us. Do I allow these energies to dominate me and determine my actions? Or by my will power can I direct these energies in ways I feel are right? In other words, does my body rule over my spirit, or does my spirit rule over my body? Conflicts arise in the heart when our sexual desires try to propel us in a direction that our judgment feels is wrong. Conflicts also arise in the world around us when we engage in sexual activities that are not socially acceptable.

The Power of Christ to Heal Sexual Compulsions

Problems related to sexuality can affect our health physically, psychologically, and even spiritually. In much of Africa, one major problem is multiple-partner heterosexual activity. This often begins during adolescence. It is one reason for the rapid spread of the HIV/AIDS epidemic in many African countries.

Large numbers of young people in the Congo and other countries of Central Africa have become Christians and have made a genuine commitment to Christ. Some of them, however, had already become involved in promiscuous heterosexual activity. Many of them have found that, even when they become Christians, they cannot break the promiscuous pattern of sexual activity to which they had already become accustomed.

A nineteen-year-old girl named Sophie came to see me in the clinic. She complained of abdominal pain, irregular monthly periods, and difficulty in concentrating on her studies. I could find no physical cause for her problems. When I inquired about her personal life, she assured me that everything was in order. She had accepted Christ two years previously and was active in the youth Bible study league of the local church. I encouraged her to talk with Mrs. Matala, and she began consulting with her. Two weeks later she and Mrs. Matala explained to me what had occurred during the times of consultation.

Mrs. Matala inquired about Sophie's physical complaints. Then she gently asked questions concerning other aspects of Sophie's life. Sophie suddenly broke down and poured out a long story of anguish and pain. She had numerous boyfriends. And although she knew it was wrong to sleep with them, she did not have the courage or the desire to refuse them. After all, some of them were in the Bible study group. She begged Mrs. Matala to help her.

Mrs. Matala understands the dynamics of this sort of behavior. Such promiscuity is not demonic, but it is enslavement to sinful behavior. In her heart Sophie knew this, but she could not set herself free. Mrs. Matala asked Sophie if she really wanted to be set free. When Sophie affirmed that she did, Mrs. Matala encouraged her to tell the whole story to Jesus, confess her sins, and ask for his forgiveness and cleansing power. She then instructed Sophie to renounce this sinful practice and, in her heart and later in her actions, to break completely her relationships with these boyfriends. Sophie was able to do all of this.

During a subsequent consultation, Mrs. Matala

asked Sophie if she would like the pastoral staff to pray with her for liberation from this bondage. Sophie said she would like that. The following day, the pastoral staff met with her and heard her story. They reassured her of her salvation, that Christ had forgiven her, and that his power could now strengthen her and protect her from immorality. As they prayed with her, they prayed against the spirit of immorality. They asked Christ to complete his work of healing Sophie's emotions, feelings, and desires. Finally, they asked the Lord to protect her completely from immorality day and night, and they committed her to his care.

Following this, Mrs. Matala outlined for Sophie how she must think and what she must do to remain free from her bondage to immorality. Follow-up since then has confirmed that, like Dr. Katele, Sophie has been set free. She is now ready to assume the responsibilities of marriage and motherhood.

Sophie is one among hundreds of men and women who have been set free from bondage to immorality. The power of Christ combined with prayer and loving counsel by pastoral and medical caregivers can bring liberation and healing to those who are bound by strong sinful behavior patterns. Incidentally, Sophie's physical complaints disappeared without medical treatment. Fortunately, her serological test for AIDS was negative. Tragically, however, for numerous other young people with similar stories, the virus has already infected them, and no cure for that has yet been found.

The Spiritual Dimension of Sexual Compulsions

The power of Christ in the heart of a person like Dr. Katele or Sophie can heal sexual compulsions and can restore health to their sexuality. But what about prevention? How can we combat the powerful influences drawing people into unhealthy compulsive sexual behaviors?

The Apostle Paul tells us that our real struggles are not against human beings but are "against the wicked spiritual forces in the heavenly world, the rulers, authorities, and cosmic powers of this dark age" (Ephesians 6:12). Because of our modern rationalistic culture, we understand this passage poorly. What are these powers? Where is the heavenly world? How do these powers act on us?

The heavenly world is the unseen spiritual realm that surrounds us and in which we live our daily lives. These rulers, authorities, and cosmic powers are spiritual forces acting in human affairs through human structures—organizations, institutions, governments, media—to deceive, corrupt, and manipulate them. The spirit of hatred operating through the Nazi government produced the Holocaust. The spirit of conflict working in many ethnic groups motivates genocidal conflicts all over the world. The spirit of immorality has engineered the sexual revolution and opened the door to physical and psychological illnesses that are destroying the lives and health of millions of people. Let me illustrate this with a story.

In 1994 I went to Kenya to visit other mission hospitals and to attend a medical conference. A dear Congolese friend and colleague, who is a Christian orthopedic surgeon, accompanied me. One evening I asked him why there was so much immorality in the Congo (formerly Zaïre). As he described what he had observed during his years of study in the university and as a medical student in Kinshasa, I was appalled.

When this doctor finished medical school, he and his wife went to Belgium, where he was to receive his orthopedic specialty training. He said the situation in Belgium was even worse than in Kinshasa. In the hospital where he was training, he was the only doctor on the surgical staff who was faithful to his wife. The other doctors and nurses often mocked him because of this.

During his years as medical director of a large mission hospital in the Congo, he made numerous administrative trips to Kinshasa. He had friends high up in the government of President Mobutu, and he visited them a couple of times in their homes. He described the overpowering sense of oppression in these wealthy homes, where numerous attractive young women were sexually available for family and friends.

I asked him how it was that the head of state himself did not seem to have contracted HIV infection. He told me that the presidential staff went to great lengths to protect him from possible exposure. That night my head was spinning because of these disturbing accounts, and I had trouble sleeping.

A week later, I was attending a medical conference in the highlands of Kenya. One Saturday evening my spirit was very troubled, and I went out to pray under the stars. In anguish I told the Lord of the many thousands of people in hundreds of intercessory groups across the land of Zaïre who had been praying for years for the liberation of their country from the oppressive hands of evildoers. My frustration was mingled with anger as I exclaimed to the Lord, "But you are silent!"

Then I pled with God about AIDS. I said, "Lord, you gave us this ministry of bringing healing to the hearts, souls, and spirits of HIV positive persons, but you are not healing their bodies. Why not? We have been pleading for you to cure them, but you are silent. Are you powerless? So many babies and young mothers—who have done no wrong—have died. Even though they have gone to heaven, who on earth praises you because their baby or their daughter is in heaven? On the contrary, the world weeps because they are gone, and how can this bring glory to you?" I leaned on the fence and wept bitterly. There was no answer.

The following afternoon I took my Bible and went for a walk in the lovely green tea fields. "Father, I have brought this book along with me, and I am going to read to you things you have written, promises you have made but are not keeping." A sudden rainshower stopped our conversation at that point and sent me running back to the lodge.

There I was reading a book on strategic prayer. The author referred to Revelation 17. This is what I read:

> Then one of the angels who had the seven bowls came to me and said, "Come, and I will show you how the famous prostitute is to be punished, that great city that is built near many rivers. The kings of the earth practiced sexual immorality with her, and the people of the world became drunk from drinking the wine of her immorality." (vv. 1-2)

I groaned in my spirit, and three words flashed across my mind: Mobutu, Zaïre, and AIDS. Then a quiet voice spoke in the depths of my being. "This is the answer to your questions. I am the Almighty God, but I cannot save Zaïre nor can I stop AIDS as long as the people of the world and their leaders choose the spirit of immorality."

After some minutes, I said, "Then Lord, what is the use? We may as well give up."

I sensed the Lord urging me to keep reading.

In chapter 17, John describes the strange symbolic beast with seven heads and ten horns. To me this represents the corrupted institutional powers that run much of the world, the political structures, industrial, financial, and commercial empires, many of the educational institutions, and the modern media, the fleshing-out of the evil powers Paul speaks of in Ephesians 6:12. John says, "They will fight against the Lamb, but the Lamb, *together with his called, chosen, and faithful followers*, will defeat them, because he is Lord of lords, and King of kings" (Revelation 17:14, italics mine). I felt the Lord saying to me, "I will not overcome these powers alone. But together with all of you, if you remain faithful, strong, and a vessel for my power, *we will overcome them*."

I realized in a new way that the battle to protect the sexual health of people requires more than physical technology, social activities, and educational campaigns. It must involve combat against the pervasive spirit of immorality that has influenced all parts of the world and every aspect of society. We must engage in concerted prayer and make a clear proclamation of God's truth as we bring people the good news of healing and teach them how we can live a healthy and fulfilling life.

The Nature of Depression

Depression is another very serious illness which assaults the core of the self. Self-affirmation is diminished, and self-confidence is shaken. Initiative and creativity are suppressed, concentration requires more and more effort, and the joy of living is gone. Fatigue increases, food loses its appeal, and illness and infections become frequent. Without adequate help, a depressed person can go into despair and become suicidal.

The causes of depression are many. Some are internal, related to a genetic predisposition or to an imbalance in minerals or hormones. External causes are multiple. There may be the loss of an important relationship—death of a spouse or child, divorce, or loss of a close friend or colleague. Life may have been disrupted by circumstances beyond the person's control, such as the loss of a job or of material resources, leading to a feeling of helplessness. A sense of failure can depress the spirit. Chronic illness or a prolonged separation from loved ones can also lead to depression.

Many books have been written about depression, its causes, and its numerous treatments. We will not duplicate those materials or analyze them. But we can safely conclude that depression is a serious problem of the heart. Recovering from depression often requires the help of qualified counselors or physicians.

All of us struggle with the discouragement that can lead to depression. Discouragement and even mild, short-term depression do not necessarily require professional help. Christ gives us resources that can restore the spirit and bring renewed peace to the heart.

Jesus' approach for one man's depression

In some ways, Simon Peter's personality set him up for assaults on his self-image. Blustering and outspoken, he was often putting his worst foot forward. He tried to walk on the water and almost drowned (Matthew 14:22-33). He opened his mouth on the Mount of Transfiguration and God himself told him to be quiet (Mark 9:2-8). Within minutes after his marvelous recognition and affirmation of Jesus' true identity, Christ had to rebuke him for listening to Satan rather than to God (Matthew 16:13-23).

As the world system closed in on Jesus, Peter's own

world crashed. On the night before Jesus' crucifixion Peter, in false humility, refused to let Jesus wash his feet, then blurted out that he needed a total body wash. Jesus rebuked him for both remarks (John 13:2-11). Peter loudly proclaimed his loyalty to Jesus even if it meant death (Mark 14:27-31) only to have Jesus tell him that soon he would deny Jesus publicly. Peter rose up in arms to defend his teacher when the crowd came to arrest Jesus, and Jesus told him that was unnecessary (John 18:10-11). Then a few hours later, like a weak child, Peter denied to three servant girls ever having known Jesus (Mark 14:66-72). At that moment, something in Peter died. He was no longer Peter, the rock; he had become once again simply Simon the fisherman. He wept bitterly.

Today one might say that Peter was in deep depression. Peter hid during the rest of Jesus' trial, crucifixion, and death. What was perhaps his worst failure was not to be present at Jesus' burial. In eastern and African cultures, it is unthinkable for family members and close friends to be absent from a funeral or burial of a loved one. Yet Peter, Jesus' trusted disciple, was absent when Jesus' body was placed in the tomb.

Peter did, however, remain with his fellow disciples and shared their confusion, fear, and depression. He and the others did see the resurrected Jesus, yet none of them could grasp the full significance of what had occurred. People in depression have trouble handling new information.

Finally, in desperation Peter returned to the only thing he knew how to do well. He had been a successful fisherman in Galilee. Peter went back there to fish, taking along several of the other fishermen-disciples. Fishing there is best at night, and Peter led his colleagues to where he knew they would find an abundant catch. All night they fished but caught nothing. Doing what he knew he could do well, Peter failed.

In this story of Peter, many elements of depression are woven together. For three years Jesus had been at the center of Peter's life. Peter had left everything to follow Jesus. Then when the world took Jesus away from Peter, Peter's inner moorings were washed away and his spirit crashed. Peter seemed caught in titanic spiritual and political forces he could not control. Repeated blows to his ego further assaulted his spirit. Finally he failed at what he thought he could always do well.

I can picture Peter in the early morning mist, slumped naked in the bow of the boat, totally discouraged. Holding his throbbing temples in his hands, he could not recognize the well-known voice of someone calling from the shore. His subconscious mind may have latched onto something familiar in the voice or in the instructions given, but it did not register in his conscious mind. However, when he heard the joyful voice of John shouting, "It's the Lord!" he grabbed his clothes, sprang out of the boat into the water, and swam furiously to shore. He fell at Jesus' feet and probably blurted out, "Lord, where in the world have you been when I needed you most?"

That would have been a most pertinent question to ask. As Peter had been getting more and more depressed, where *had* Jesus been? Did he not know that his trusted disciple was in deep suffering and despair?

Yes, Jesus knew, and he was waiting for the right moment. While waiting, and even while carrying the sins of the whole world in his own body, Jesus had been praying for Peter (Luke 22:31-32). Jesus had followed Peter to Galilee. He knew where he was, sensed what he was going through, and in the right moment he came to find him.

Here on the shore of Galilee Jesus returned to Peter and to the center of his life. He took him aside, not to rebuke him for his denial but to heal him. Jesus reaffirmed Peter as a person. Three times he asked Peter if he loved him, and three times Peter declared that he did. In this way, Jesus led Peter to speak a word to the depths of his own heart, namely, that Jesus was once again his first love and the center of his life. And Peter spoke that word to himself in the presence of Jesus.

There is no more powerful therapy for depression than the presence of the living Jesus in the depths of a broken heart. When a depressed person can say in his heart, "Jesus, I love you," healing can begin. This does not necessarily replace other treatments, but it begins the process of rebuilding the self-image around the mighty presence of Jesus in the heart. When Jesus is in the heart of a depressed person, self-affirmation follows and healing can come.

Jesus then added something else to his therapy. He put Peter to work, reaffirming the immense task he had given to Peter to build his church and to care for others. This gave Peter a reason to go on living. It renewed his sense of responsibility and reassured him that he was still useful to Jesus.

The final step in Peter's rehabilitation took place some days later. Jesus was now gone from Peter's physical life, but the Holy Spirit came to Peter's whole self on the day of Pentecost. Then Peter was healed and empowered. Instead of the power and position he might have chosen, Peter would experience persecution, sacrifice, and eventual martyrdom. Peter was ready for all of this because Jesus, through the Holy Spirit, now filled Peter's whole being.

Spiritual help with depression

Christians as well as non-Christians suffer depression. I

know, for I have been depressed myself. Time after time in my medical service, circumstances have threatened to undo the work God has given us to do in Africa. Many times I could see no way out and cried out in anguish, "My God, why have you forsaken me?" I knew I was depressed when my sense of humor disappeared, my appetite left, and I no longer had any joy in living.

In times like those, I would turn to the Psalms.

> The Lord is my light and my salvation. Whom shall I fear? (Psalm 27:1, KJV)

> My help comes from the Lord who made heaven and earth. (Psalm 121:2, KJV)

> I will always thank the Lord; I will never stop praising him. (Psalm 34:1, TEV).

But how can you praise the Lord when you are depressed?

Sometimes I would literally have to force myself to praise the Lord. It would be a battle between my will and all of my feelings and emotions. When by a conscious decision I mouthed words of praise to God, the presence of the Lord permeated the depths of my spirit. Often the struggle would continue for days or even weeks, but if I remained faithful in praising God and seeking him, Jesus would clothe me in a garment of praise and remove the spirit of heaviness (Isaiah 61:3, KJV). My strength, appetite, and sense of humor would return, and I could go on in the strength of the Lord. Jesus and God's Word can be of great help in healing depression and returning a person to creative life.

Caregiver help with depression

When discouragement comes, and even early depression, the Lord is an ever-present help in the time of need. If, however, the depression progresses, we should turn in faith to those trained to care for people with this condition. As the Spirit of God comes alongside to help us, so can caregivers who are able to bring the Lord into the healing process. Walking through a dark valley without help can be dangerous. Coming to a caregiver for guidance, wisdom, and encouragement can bring light into the darkness. It can help show the way toward renewal of mind and of spirit.[2]

Seeking help is not a sign of weakness; it is a sign of maturity. God has created us to live in relationships of interdependence with others. If I am to serve others as God would have me to, I also need to be able to accept the help of others and even, in time of need, to seek that help.

When we are discouraged, the limits of our abilities become evident. We cannot do what we would like to do or feel we should do. This should bring important questions into focus: Are my goals real? Are they achievable? Or do they need to be re-examined?

Such times call for developing a more intimate relationship with our Creator. Depression can lead us to seek God more seriously and trust him more earnestly. Depression will also bring us to cry out desperately for help. Isaiah cried, "Seek the Lord while he may be found; call upon him while he is near" (Isaiah 55:6, NIV).

10

The Power of Forgiveness

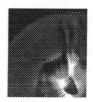

We have seen how Christ can help us with many of our heart problems and that this can help us better cope with physical diseases. We must now be more radical and come to grips with the sin or sins underlying these problems.

Jesus and the Paralyzed Man

The second chapter of Mark gives a fascinating account of the forgiveness of sin and the healing of a physical disability.

> A few days later Jesus went back to Capernaum, and the news spread that he was at home. So many people came together that there was no room left, not even out in front of the door. Jesus was preaching the message to them when four men arrived, carrying a paralyzed man to Jesus. Because of the crowd, however, they could not get

the man to him. So they made a hole in the roof right above the place where Jesus was. When they had made an opening, they let the man down, lying on his mat. Seeing how much faith they had, Jesus said to the paralyzed man, "My son, your sins are forgiven."

Some teachers of the Law who were sitting there thought to themselves, "How does he dare talk like this? This is blasphemy! God is the only one who can forgive sins!"

At once Jesus knew what they were thinking, so he said to them, "Why do you think such things? Is it easier to say to this paralyzed man, 'Your sins are forgiven,' or to say, 'Get up, pick up your mat, and walk'? I will prove to you, then, that the Son of Man has authority on earth to forgive sins." So he said to the paralyzed man, "I tell you, get up, pick up your mat, and go home!"

While they all watched, the man got up, picked up his mat, and hurried away. They were all completely amazed and praised God, saying, "We have never seen anything like this!" (Mark 2:1-12)

On several occasions Jesus dealt with sin when he healed sick persons. This account in Mark, however, is the only one in which Jesus forgave sin prior to healing the person of the physical problem. What can we learn from this?

One significant factor is the ease with which Jesus integrated the various aspects of his ministry. He was in the middle of preaching when he was confronted with this person in need of healing. For Jesus, it was natural to move immediately from preaching to healing. This was an abrupt and almost brutal interrup-

tion. Suddenly there was a clatter overhead as men removed tiles from the roof. Then dust came cascading
down on Jesus and those near him. What a mess! In
such a situation I would have been furious, but Jesus
was undisturbed. He considered this not an interruption but rather an opportunity to help and to teach.
Jesus did not divide his life and ministry into separate
categories but fit them all together in harmony.

Jesus observed the whole group who came to present this need. They may have been men of the sick
man's family. Jesus saw their concern, their initiative,
their persistence in spite of obstacles, and their faith
in his ability to help their friend or family member.
Jesus was favorably impressed, and he responded with
compassion. Jesus treated the whole family, and we, as
caregivers, must do the same. We must not separate
the sick person from those who care for him.

Jesus' first word to the suffering man was a word of
affirmation. He addressed him as "My son." This was
not paternalism but compassion, not condescension
but love. It was intentional; Jesus probably detected in
the paralyzed man the wounds of rejection or alienation. This salutation was the beginning of the man's
healing.

Did Jesus suspect that the paralysis came from a sin
in this man's life? It is possible that he did, and there
could indeed be such a connection. This could have
been a case of hysterical paralysis due to some serious
sin, conflict, or psychological trauma. Or the inability
to walk could have been the physical consequence of a
deep-seated heart problem.

I believe that Jesus perceived in this young man's
heart a deep problem related to a particular sin in his
life that had precipitated a physical disorder leading
to his inability to walk. Without wasting time, Jesus
went to the deep roots of the man's problem by deal-

ing with the remorse, shame, or fear entrenched in his heart. However, the record does not say what Jesus perceived. We simply know that, with this particular person, he chose to begin with forgiveness as his initial therapeutic measure. What can we conclude from this?

Sin and sickness are interrelated, either directly or indirectly. Jesus knew this. He understood how physical problems, social relationships, and psychological and spiritual issues all mesh and are parts of the whole picture. He shows us here that forgiveness of sin can have a powerful physical healing effect. Jesus wanted to show to this man, to his audience, and to all of us the therapeutic power of forgiveness.

Forgiveness and Healing

When we confess our sin, we are recognizing the reality of personal sin, accepting responsibility for it, and deciding to turn away from it. When the assurance of forgiveness comes, it can remove the guilt, fear, and shame of sin, and defuse the tension and stresses caused by it. The immune system is then released from the suppressive effects of these negative feelings and emotions, and healing can occur.

How all of this came together in the case of the paralyzed man, we do not know. We don't have all the details. The physical healing may have been miraculous, beyond explanation by the scientific principles we know. Or it may have resulted from the resolution of serious psycho-spiritual problems in this man's life, which then removed whatever was causing his disability. Whatever the actual process was, we do know that Jesus associated forgiveness with healing.

The teachers of the Law were correct in questioning Jesus' authority to forgive sin. In the Jewish faith, forgiveness came only when the prescribed blood sacrifice was properly performed at the Temple in Jerusalem. The priest himself could not forgive sin. He could only assure repentant persons that God had forgiven them when they had brought the proper sacrifice.

The teachers of the Law were nevertheless in error in ascribing blasphemy to Jesus because they did not know that something new had happened: God had come into their midst in Jesus Christ. Jesus had the authority to forgive sin because he was God in the flesh. Furthermore, sacrifices were no longer necessary because Jesus himself was about to make the complete and final sacrifice for sin.

Jesus Alone Can Forgive

I cannot forgive another person's sin or sins. I can of course forgive someone who has wronged me. Beyond that I have no authority to forgive sin—as a physician, a counselor, or a Christian. Neither can we accuse a sick person of having sinned. What we can do, however, is to help a person identify the sin or sins that need to be confessed to Jesus. This requires much gentleness, tact, and compassion. It is best done by careful questioning and by using Scripture, remembering that it is only the sick person who can make this confession and only Jesus who can forgive.

Jesus himself did not accuse anyone of sin. He ate with but did not accuse Zaccheus, who had been deeply involved in corruption and had robbed many people. Just being in the presence of Jesus helped Zaccheus see his own sinfulness and need for repentance (Luke 19:1-10). Jesus did not accuse the tax-collector in the Temple, but he made it clear that this man had received the mercy for which he was praying (Luke 18:9-14).

Although we do not have the authority to forgive

someone's sin, we do have the authority and the wonderful privilege of assuring a person of God's forgiveness when the person has confessed those sins to Christ. This is what is called the word of absolution, and it declares—on the authority of Christ—that a person has been forgiven. This word has great healing power. Our authority to give a word of absolution is based on what Jesus said to this paralyzed man and to the teachers of the Law who witnessed it. It is also based on what John declared, "If we confess our sins to God, he will keep his promise and do what is right. He will forgive us our sins and purify us from all our wrong doing" (1 John 1:9).

Jesus alone can forgive sins. Since medicine, psychology, and even the church have no authority to forgive sins, this is why faith in Christ is crucial for the healing of the wounds of sin, of a spirit broken by guilt, and of a contrite heart.

Hepatitis B, Confession, and Healing

I described in chapter 6 my illness when I was suffering from hepatitis B. I realized my own personal involvement in that disease process, for I had been abusing my body by overwork. I was not just a "victim" of hepatitis B but was also an active part of the process of the illness. My own personal attitudes and behavior were aggravating my illness. I had been living sinfully by refusing the God-ordained weekly rest from the press of duties. For me as a physician, taking Sundays off was seldom possible. Nevertheless, this did not absolve me from the command of taking equivalent time for rest and for physical and spiritual refreshment. I was sinning against God, against myself, and against my family and associates. I was in need of forgiveness.

When I was confronted with my sinful behavior, I immediately confessed this to God and had the assurance of forgiveness. I also received the imperative to stop sinning; in other words, I had to get my behavior in order. With the help of my wife and my colleagues, I made a serious effort to do that. As a result, I began taking time not only for rest but for reflection and for communication with others and with God himself. This was the beginning of my healing.

As I reflected, I began to examine other aspects of my life, of my relationships, and of my work. Were there other problems to be resolved, other areas of my life and thoughts that needed restoration?

From this I learned that illness, whatever its nature, can be a marvelous school, an opportunity to learn new things about life, about self, and about the world. I discovered many other things in my life that needed confession, repentance (turning away from), and forgiveness. I brought these to the Lord to leave them in his hands once and for all. Miriam and I talked at length about many aspects of our life together in order to heal problems between us. I sought the counsel of others, for the wise counsel of spiritually mature people can be of great value.

During this process of reflection and learning in the summer of 1987, I had a needle biopsy of my liver. The results showed early cirrhosis of the liver, with my liver cells full of the DNA of the hepatitis B virus. I continued my reflections, tried to eat a balanced diet, and prayed much. Many others prayed for me and with me. In early 1988 I signed in as a participant in an experimental treatment trial testing a new and as yet unconfirmed therapy for hepatitis B. The trial team drew my blood to check various parameters of the infection. Two weeks later the physician in charge called me on the phone to say that I did not qualify for this treatment trial. They could not find any evidence of hepatitis B in my blood!

Oh me of little faith, I assumed that a mistake had been made, and I insisted they test my blood again. When the second result confirmed the first, it became clear to my heart: God had indeed healed me and my hepatitis B was gone. I then turned to him to thank him for what he had done. I also thanked him for the many people who had prayed for me, and who by their counsel and support had encouraged me to participate with God in this healing process. Recognition and confession of my sin, the forgiveness of Christ, and turning from my sinful and unhealthy behavior contributed much to the elimination of the hepatitis B virus and the healing of my liver. So also did the prayers, concern, and encouragement of family and friends, for a compassionate caring community has great therapeutic power.

We are not victims of illness, even of accidents. Yes, they do happen to us, but once they happen, we become participants in the process, either active participants or passive recipients. Self-examination is part of the active participation we need to make. That examination may reveal problems we need to solve, thoughts or behavior we need to change, or sins we must confess. When we do what needs to be done, we participate in our own healing process. The assurance of forgiveness, of restoration of relationships, and of cleansing from the inner wounds removes the heart problems depressing our recuperative powers. This is how the forgiveness of sin has such a powerful healing effect.

The Progression of Healing

David, the magnificent singing king of Israel, had marvelous God-given insight into this healing process.

In Psalm 103 he outlines the fascinating progression that can take place from the darkness and despair of illness to glorious health. This is what he says:

> Praise the Lord, my soul! All my being, praise
> his holy name!
> Praise the Lord, my soul, and do not forget
> how kind he is.
> He forgives all my sins and heals all my dis-
> eases.
> He keeps me from the grave and blesses me
> with love and mercy.
> He fills my life with good things, so that I
> stay young and strong like an eagle. (Psalm
> 103:1-5)

Let's look at the progression in this hymn.

David starts with praise to God
In another psalm he says, "Every face turned toward him grows brighter" (Psalm 34:5, JB). Praising God lifts our view from ourselves, our troubles, or our hepatitis, chronic fatigue syndrome, cancer, or high blood pressure to God himself. In praise we concentrate on the goodness of God and what he has done. This can bring joy into the thoughts, feelings, and emotions, and this joy can strengthen the immune system. Praise is good for our health!

David reflects on what God has done for him
In spite of the most horrible circumstances in which we may find ourselves (and David himself got into many frightful messes), we can always identify something that shows the goodness of God. Putting our thoughts on that, however small it may be, can lift our spirits from the darkness of despair to a tiny point of

light and hope. This again can strengthen our recuperative powers.

David recognizes that forgiveness of sin leads to healing of disease

From his own experience, David was deeply aware of how the forgiveness of sin brings new life and renewed physical strength. He wrote two psalms about this—Psalm 32 and Psalm 51. I've learned that the confession of sins that have nothing whatsoever to do with the illness is also therapeutic. Confession opens the "rooms" of the heart to Jesus, the great "Heart Cleaner," making room for his peace and joy.

David sees despair and the fear of death as affecting health and recuperative powers

Deliverance from despair and from the fear of the grave comes from God as we permit him to lead us through the above steps, and as we respond to what he is in the process of doing. God will not exempt us from physical death, for we all will eventually die. But God can take away the frightful weight of the fear of death, thus freeing us in the meantime for fullness of life.

David receives blessings and mercy from God

The word blessing means happiness. When our minds are turned toward God, when we reflect on what he has done, and when we receive forgiveness and the healing of heart, mind, and spirit with deliverance from the fear of death, all kinds of good and happy things can occur. We begin noticing the intricate design at the center of a flower, the wonderful scent of newly mown grass, the mood-lifting power of music, and the smiles of family and friends. The eyes and ears of our heart are opened to the beauties and delights of life as we are set free from the darkness of despair.

David accepts the health and strength God provides
Such a song of confession and praise leads to health of mind, heart, and spirit. By strengthening the recuperative powers of the body, it can often lead to increased strength. In many cases (though not all) it can even lead to complete physical healing. Once again we can feel "young and strong like an eagle."

The Serpent in the Wilderness

There is a story in the Old Testament that has often disturbed me. It is in chapter 21 in the book of Numbers. The children of Israel had grown impatient with the length of their trip to the Promised Land and the difficulties they were experiencing. They began to grumble and complain. So, God sent snakes to their camp that bit many people, and those who were bitten died. The people recognized their bad attitude and behavior and asked Moses to pray to God to forgive them and take the snakes away. God told Moses to make a bronze snake and put it on a tall pole in the middle of the camp where everyone could see it. Then when anyone was bitten and looked at this bronze serpent, he or she would not die.

Miriam and I have served for many years in Africa. In African culture, fetishes, charms, and idols are very important, for in the thinking of the people, they possess magical power. They can protect us from illness, can heal many diseases, and can ward off evil spirits. We have tried to help people realize that our real help comes from God and that we do not need to depend on charms or magical practices.

This story has disturbed me because the bronze serpent seemed to me to be a fetish, something which, when we look at it, would have power to heal. Now, however, I recognize the real significance of this story.

Its meaning is so important that Jesus, in his evening conversation with Nicodemus recorded in John chapter 3, compared this incident with what he soon would do on the cross.

Israel had sinned against God by grumbling and complaining. They were suffering the consequences of this sin, consequences in the form of venomous serpents. Moses put the bronze serpent on the pole, not as a fetish with magical powers but as the symbol of the sin of the people. They had to look on the symbol of their own sin of complaining, recognize it as sin, and accept responsibility for it in order to be healed. The bronze serpent had no magical power to heal. It was what took place in the mind and heart of the person bitten that accomplished the healing.

Here then is true confession.

Confession is looking at our own sin and seeing it as rebellion

My illness with hepatitis B showed me that I was depending on my own strength and not on God. I was making my own decisions, and I had to acknowledge that. My real problem was my attitude of independence, and it was manifesting itself in my unhealthy behavior. My overwork had been abusing the body God has given me, and I had to admit to myself and to God I was doing wrong. My "serpent" was workaholism, which I was rationalizing as "serving God by helping others."

Confession is bringing our rebellion and our wrongdoing to Jesus, telling him we have done wrong and are sorry

Our sorrow must be because we have done wrong to him, disobeyed him, and grieved him. We have left him out of a vital part of our lives. This sorrow must not be simply because of the consequences we are suffering from our wrongdoing. I was sorry not just because my liver was inflamed, but because I was not taking my directions from Jesus. I was ignoring him and doing my own thing.

Confession is asking for forgiveness
We must ask for forgiveness, and when we do, it will never be denied. There is no question about it; God forgives, for that is his business.

We must accept our forgiveness and the purifying power of God in our hearts
He will indeed purify the "bent" of our hearts for that wrongdoing. This purification may be immediate, or it may take time, but it will happen.

We must turn away from that sin, rejecting it completely and embracing a new way
That is what the word repentance means. God's forgiveness of my workaholic lifestyle would have been of minimal benefit to me had I not, by my conscious decision, chosen to adopt a new pattern of living.

John wrote, "As Moses lifted up the serpent on a pole in the desert, in the same way the Son of Man must be lifted up, so that everyone who believes in him may have eternal life" (John 3:14-15). Jesus was lifted up on a tree when he had taken our sin into himself. When I looked at Jesus on the cross, I saw that he had taken into his own body my workaholism, my rationalization, and my pride. I recognized and acknowledged that my sins were part of the human sin that had put him on the cross. I confessed my sins to him and asked for his forgiveness. I then made my decision to turn from them. I knew he had forgiven me, and that healed my guilt. I knew also that he overcame the enslaving power of these sins by rising from death, so my heart understood that I had been set free. Then my immune system was able to eliminate the virus, and my liver recovered. Forgiveness has great power to heal.

Heart Cleaning Applied

What makes "heart cleaning" by Christ so powerful and unique is this: Christ listens to us whenever we want to talk to him. If Christ is already present in your heart, you can converse with him freely and frankly at any time, day or night. He has no office hours, nor does he have a fee schedule. If you have not invited Christ to enter your heart, he is nevertheless waiting to hear your call for help, healing, and liberation. When you ask him to come and live within your spirit, he will do so and will make his healing resources available to you.

We have been discussing some of the deep hurts of the soul, the pain, the wounds, and the heartaches that are a part of the life of all of us. Now imagine Christ standing in front of you holding in one hand an enormous open garbage bucket and in the other hand a voluminous bottle of healing balm.

If your heart problem is fear, describe this fear to him. Pour into his bucket the whole story of your fears and the events that have brought them into your life. Then imagine him putting the lid on the bucket so you will see those fears no more. Now expose the wounds in your heart made by those events and fears and ask Jesus to pour his healing balm on them. The events that caused your fears may not disappear from your memory, but the pain associated with them will be gone. Your spirit will now know that, if or when these memories recur, Jesus is standing with you and that "there is nothing in all creation that will ever be able to separate us from the love of God which is ours through Jesus Christ our Lord" (Romans 8:39).

If your heartache is a broken relationship, or anger, or guilt, or distressing sexual behavior, or addiction to tobacco or alcohol, or depression, or all of the above, or anything else, the garbage bucket of Christ is sufficient to contain it all, and his healing balm will never run dry.

Christ heals the broken heart and the wounded spirit, but he can do so only when we bring our brokenness to him. You can do this alone, in the quietness of your room, in a chapel or church, or in a secluded spot in the beauties of nature. Let your tears flow freely, for tears themselves have a healing effect. Remember that Christ died for our tears (Isaiah 53:4).

Confession can also be done as part of a healing community. Although this may seem threatening, in reality it can be highly beneficial. In the New Testament James tells us, "Confess your sins to one another and pray for one another, so that you will be healed. The prayer of a good person has a powerful effect" (James 5:16). In such a healing community, the sharing of problems, hurts, and sins can bring the realization that our own problems are not unique. Insights shared by others who have wrestled with similar problems can provide new wisdom. The power of prayer in community multiplies as many words of healing can be spoken by members of the group.

Identifying and articulating the deep aches of the heart can be difficult. We may need the help of a wise advocate to facilitate our own understanding of these heart problems and to encourage us to "dump them into Christ's garbage bucket." By whatever process seems best, whether alone, within a caring community, or with a wise counselor, we can safely bring our hurts, our cares, and our sins to the Healer, knowing that he does indeed care for us.

11

Illness: Tragedy or Challenge?

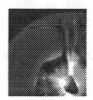

We often consider diseases, disasters, and accidents as tragedies. They threaten us, impose unwanted changes on our way of life, and disturb our inner equilibrium. What we do with the disease, disaster, or accident, however, can be something else. We do have a choice. We can think of these trials as tragedies and of ourselves as victims. While this outlook is logical enough, its message to the heart won't help us cope. When the heart accepts victim status, it will send doleful messages to the body's defense systems, which will then, at best, engage only in a holding operation.

But if the heart can say, "I wish this hadn't happened to me, but it has. Now what can I do to make something good out of it?" this sends a different message to the body's systems: "Mobilize!"

Effective mobilization requires resources. Let's review the resources available to us and see how we can apply them when illness comes. These resources are useful even when we face a life-threatening or debilitating physical disease.

Physical Resources

Medical care

Medicine and medical care in all its forms bring to us a panorama of diagnostic and therapeutic technologies. These technologies are gifts from God because they are the fleshing-out of the creative abilities God has put within us. They are also our growing but limited response to God's command to study life and to be co-managers of nature with him.

We are not denying faith in God when we use what God has given us. On the contrary, refusing to take needed medicine is refusing to take what God has enabled us to discover and develop. Can God help us when we refuse the help he has already provided through human wisdom and creativity?

Consulting a physician or other health care professional early in the course of an illness is so important. We gain nothing by temporizing. Adequate diagnostic examinations are necessary to bring into focus the causes of the problem.

Nevertheless, we need to remember that even the best medical care is only a part of the healing process. Medicine helps, and it is often essential, but it is our own recuperative powers that make us well.

The immune system

We have our own built-in immune system, and we talked about this in chapter 4. We now know there are things we can do to strengthen the immune system so it can better cope with whatever the disease may be.

Nutrition. Nutritional deficiencies open the door to many diseases. Nutritional sufficiencies can reinforce the immune system by providing the basic raw materials the body needs to make white blood cells, antibodies, and the other complex proteins and chemicals we need to fight disease.

Eating three good meals a day, with a diet rich in fiber and vitamins, moderate in carbohydrates and proteins, and low in animal fats, makes excellent health sense. The best medicine in the world, which has been available without a doctor's prescription from the very beginning, is water. Keeping water flowing in adequate quantities through the body is beneficial to health, yet most of us drink far too little. Six to ten glasses of water a day (depending on physical activity) is minimal for maintaining a healthy inner equilibrium. An adequate quantity of fluid intake is likewise a major help in overcoming many diseases.

Unfortunately the nature of many infections, including hepatitis, various fevers, and HIV/AIDS, as well as malignant diseases is such that good nutrition and adequate fluid intake can become difficult to maintain. During such times it requires effort, discipline, and the creative preparation of attractive and balanced meals. Nutritional supplements may be of some help, particularly in certain diseases. In general, however, what we receive in well-prepared meals using a variety of foods is the best source of the materials the body needs.

Prevention. We know that certain substances are harmful to the body—tobacco, certain drugs, and excessive quantities of caffeine, alcohol, salt, and calories. Avoiding harmful substances and eating with moderation make good health sense.

It also makes sense to avoid infections as much as possible, especially when one is already ill. Every infection presents a challenge to the immune system and can weaken it. Vaccinations can protect us from a variety of infections, and we should take full advantage of them. Staying away as much as possible from offending organisms can spare the immune system of unnecessary challenges. Early and effective treatment of any infection that does come is important.

Psychological Resources

We return to that marvelous verse in the book of Proverbs: "Peace of mind makes the body healthy" (Proverbs 14:30). Peace of mind does not resolve all of our problems, nor does it cure all of our physical diseases. But it does create a favorable internal environment that enables us to cope at maximum efficiency with the disease, whatever it may be. How can we find the inner peace that reinforces the body?

Remember that you are more than the part of you that is ill

When I examine sick persons, I sense that many of them have stress, worry, or inner conflicts that are affecting the illness and the person's recuperative powers. When I suggest to them the benefits of talking with a counselor, some of them become incensed. "Are you telling me my sickness is all in my head?"

But I point out to them, "*You* are sick. Head, heart, mind, and spirit are involved as well as your body, and all work together to help and strengthen one another. Working with 'heart doctors' (counselors) as well as with 'body doctors' can help you recover more quickly as a whole person." We must not forget that we are more than just our diseased or ill body.

Take the initiative

The process of healing needs to involve the one who is sick. As a physician I cannot heal you when you are ill; I can only help. Even God does not heal us without our consent because he has chosen not to impose his will upon us. Nor can God and I together heal you without your active participation in the process. Here is an example from the Bible.

A wealthy Syrian military leader named Naaman had leprosy. He had heard about a prophet in Israel named Elisha who could cure leprosy. So he made the long arduous journey from Damascus to Samaria in Israel to get help from Elisha. To his dismay, Elisha would not even come out of his house to treat him. Elisha simply sent his servant out to tell Naaman to make another difficult trip. He must drive for two days—close to forty miles—on a rough road that descended more than four thousand feet in order to wash himself seven times in the muddy Jordan River. Naaman became hopping mad at Elisha for being so rude as to refuse even to come out and see him. It was only with great reluctance that he finally accepted his own responsibility in the healing process and did as he was instructed. Had he not done so, he probably would not have been cured of his leprosy (2 Kings 5:1-14).

It is crucial to our healing for us to accept the responsibility for doing whatever it takes to get well. Many of us have a strong tendency to put the entire responsibility on the physician, other caregivers, or the health care system. Naaman insisted that Elisha come out to him, call on the name of the Lord, and wave his hand over the spots of leprosy to make him well. Many who are sick plead with me, "Doctor, please take your scalpel and cut it all out. You are the one who can make me well!"

Dr. Bernie Siegel reports that cancer patients who enter into the decision-making process about their treatment often do surprisingly well. In fact, the more "difficult" patients they are—the more questions they ask, and the more they argue—the better they do. They are the "fighters," and many of them outlive their prognosis and a few even conquer their disease. On the contrary, those who simply say, "Doctor, I'll do whatever you say, for you know best," succumb quite predictably to their malignancy.[1]

Our current culture glorifies medical and surgical technology. It promotes the illusion that medicines are essential for health and healing. The pharmaceutical industry fills our TV screens and magazines with the message that there is a pill for every pain (especially their brand-name pill!) and a medicine for every symptom. Consequently, rather than taking a hard look at what may be deep moral and spiritual factors in the illness, we grasp eagerly at whatever technical and pharmacological remedies are available. Instead of seeking to find and deal with personal causes of the pain, anxiety, or high blood pressure, we consume pills to suppress them. We want technology to attack the disease-producing elements without our being willing to deal with their causes.

Of course it's essential to have faith in the physician and other caregivers. But dumping the whole responsibility for healing on people, pills, procedures, and products will not help us. Nor should we insist that God miraculously heal us while we refuse to accept our own responsibilities in the plan of action for our recovery.

Finding out about the disease and the possible options enables a sick person to participate in treatment and recovery. Read books and articles about the disease. Don't hesitate to ask questions of your caregivers. They know much about the physical aspects of diseases and treatments. Only you know about your life. Therefore, treatment planning that takes into consideration both the technical aspects and your personal concerns can often lead to better results and more rapid recovery.

Be aware that healing is a triangular process
Healing has three sides: it involves us, a whole spectrum of caregivers, and God.

1. When I am ill, I must be involved in my own healing. This requires

- the will to live
- a decision to do what needs to be done
- the courage to act and to be persistent

After Naaman had bathed six times in the Jordan River, he still had leprosy. Only when he persisted to the end of his required course of action was he cured of his disease.

2. Caregivers can contribute much to our healing. The diagnostic and therapeutic help of family members, friends, therapists, pastors or priests, and health care providers is invaluable. So also are medicines and technical procedures, some of which attack the disease directly, while others strengthen the recuperative powers of the body.

3. God is always involved—directly or indirectly—in our healing. It is the defensive and recuperative powers God has put within us that accomplish the work of healing. A surgeon can cut open, cut out, and stitch up again, but it is our God-given mechanisms of cellular and tissue repair that heal the incision inside and out. Furthermore, when I choose to ask God to work with me in my journey toward healing, he can become involved in more than just a general sense. His power can then work in my thoughts, feelings, and spirit to bring healing and peace. His power can likewise work in my body. On some occasions God will work immediately in ways we deem miraculous. On most occasions, his power will work more slowly, in parallel with and complementing normal physiological processes to expedite healing.

An approach to healing that excludes any one of the three parts will be inadequate and may not succeed. Believing in God and determining to recover, while rejecting the help of medicine and caregivers, often fails. Many people can and do recover by making use of caregiving resources and by being very proactive themselves without any apparent faith in God. But they often fail to realize that God is indeed involved, for ultimately, regardless of our personal orientation toward spirituality, God is the Healer. Furthermore, failure to bring the spiritual factor into the healing process renders the recovery incomplete, for the spirit is not restored. Soul and body try to cope alone with the illness without the benefit either of one's own spirit or the healing resources of God.

Take stock of life

A disease is a threat to life. To cope with that threat, we need to take stock of our own situation—our assets and liabilities. What resources are available to fight this problem? What liabilities are impeding recovery? Illness requires that we take inventory.

Some years ago I had to make a hurried trip in a pick-up truck over bumpy dirt roads to the district capital. I went to ask the district medical officer to come and help us with an urgent administrative problem. We drove back in a torrential rain. I was squeezed in the cab between the government doctor and the door, each of us with a child on our lap. The next morning I awoke feeling as if I had fire down my whole left leg. An intervertebral disk had ruptured and was pressing on my left sciatic nerve like a hot poker. Nothing I did would relieve the pain. Finally, after struggling against the pain for two weeks, I submitted to the prescribed treatment: three weeks flat on my back in traction, with the foot of the bed elevated. Was this a tragedy or a challenge? In spite of the uncomfortable downhill position, I decided to make it a challenge.

All during our years in Africa, our home was on the bank of a magnificent river, the Kwilu River. Swimming, picnics with the family, and even water skiing would restore my soul after long days of work. While I lay on my back, I meditated. I thought of my life as a river like the Kwilu, and as I reviewed it, I learned a lot about myself.

Every river commences as a tiny stream, originating from a spring. As the stream twists and turns down a valley, other little streams join it, adding water to it. The stream grows into a river and more streams and rivers join it as tributaries, bringing their water into the main river. Some of this water is clean; some tributaries can be muddy or polluted.

I thought about the many streams that had come into my life. My parents were the original ones; what kind of water did they provide for me as my heritage and then through all my early years? Childhood friends, school and schoolmates, church, and the community all had important influence, most good but not all. The university, medical school, and further training also brought more "water" into my life. Marriage, children, a new country, work, and service added much more.

Some unpleasant experiences had occurred also, and dirty water had come into my life. I then wondered how much of that dirt was still mixed in the waters of my soul and how it was still affecting me. What could I do about it now?

Some of these problems I could deal with myself. Others I was able to talk over with Miriam or with a close friend. Still others I brought to the Lord. I was already aware that Jesus could heal the broken heart and the wounded spirit, and that he could help me deal with painful places in my life. So I talked to him.

For a few of the difficult scenarios of my life, I took paper and wrote them down. Then I presented them to the Lord, asking him to heal those painful areas. I envisaged what he had done in Gethsemane and on the cross and I asked him to apply his blood to those painful, dirty areas of my life. The Bible says that the blood of Christ purifies our hearts, so I drew a cross over what I had written. This told my heart that Jesus had included the sin, guilt, and pain of these experiences in the burden he carried to the cross. When I had finished talking each problem over with Jesus, I tore up the paper. This was a symbolic act that my heart could understand as meaning "the problem is now healed."

David the psalmist provides an example of this process. In Psalm 139 he goes through a long self-examination. Then he declares, "Search me, O God, and know my heart; test me and know my anxious thoughts. See if there is any offense in me, and lead me in the way everlasting" (Psalm 139:23-24, NIV).

Through those three weeks of bed rest and traction, the pain in my back disappeared. At the same time my spirit grew. I had found once again that illness can act like a schoolmaster, providing the challenge to learn new things about life. I cannot say that the recovery of my ruptured disk was related to my spiritual growth. But it provided the time and the setting for the spiritual growth to occur.

Self-examination can be painful; it likewise can be dangerous. Where there has been much trauma or abuse in previous years, the wounds of the heart will require the help of a caregiver skilled in helping people work through these serious problems. When we catch a cold or get the flu, we seldom need a physician. We can probably do all that is necessary to assure our own recovery. When appendicitis comes, however, no one would even think of trying to remove his or her own appendix. In the same way, deep problems of the heart will often require outside help. A compassionate caregiver, especially one who is familiar with the power of God, can give us much needed help in performing "surgery of the soul."

Have a merry heart

A sense of humor is the ability to perceive and enjoy the incongruities of life. Life is full of them; we can either be disturbed by them or find amusement in them. In almost every circumstance, if we exercise our imagination, we can find something incongruous (funny) and be amused by it. Laughter can then relieve the stress of the incongruity. Ancient wisdom and modern science come to the same conclusion. "A merry heart doeth good like a medicine" (Proverbs 17:22, KJV). In modern terms, laughter and joy strengthen the immune system.

In chapter 4 I referred to Norman Cousins and how he used comic movies, jokes, and funny stories to stimulate laughter. The resulting production of pleasure-giving opioids by his brain relieved his pain for up to two hours. It obviously strengthened his immune system because he recovered. Even when we perceive no humor in our own situation, a wealth of humor is available to us in books, magazines, and videos. We just have to look for it and determine to benefit from it.

Much humor is more personal. We see something funny in our circumstances and comment on it. This is the source of "one-liners" and spontaneous puns. During my residency, when I was earning fifty dollars a month, I went to buy a valentine card for Miriam. We were not yet engaged. I found a hilarious one, but it cost twenty-five cents. Was she really worth that much? So I left it in the store. When I was two blocks away and still laughing, I decided we needed that humor. The front of the card showed a shining aluminum kitchen garbage disposal with a silly grinning dog at the side wagging his tail furiously. Inside were the words: "I'm at your disposal." I was, and still am. Every time we revisit that card, I believe our immune systems get a bit stronger.

So many times humor has saved stressful situations in my medical work. In a tense meeting, a laughter-producing comment would melt the anger of an emotional conflict and allow reason to take over. Often our operating room would ring with laughter, not as a distraction but rather as a way to restore calmness to a stressful procedure. Laughter is indeed good medicine, for it has physiological as well as psychological benefits.

Emphasize pleasant experiences

Joyful times with family and friends strengthen the heart. Quiet walks out in nature—the woods, by lakes or streams, on a beach, or wherever we find God's beauty—can rejuvenate us.

Good books, art, and beautiful flowers, by stimulating creative imagination, can diminish stress. They provide momentary but real access to a new world and temporary relief from the distresses of the current situation. Whatever produces joy, creative imagination, and inner peace can help the brain produce neurochemicals that reinforce the physical response to disease.

Music can bring about relaxation. It can do even more than that. It speaks to the deep mind, calling forth positive memories and stimulating constructive reflections. Music therapy has positive physiological benefits. Neurochemicals stimulated by Beethoven's sixth symphony, Dvorak's New World symphony, and Bach's organ toccatas and fugues increase my immunity. Handel's Water Music suite and John Philip Sousa's marches set my white blood cells to dancing.[2]

Make a worry list

Worry is extremely effective at stealing peace of mind. Worries are a part of our human condition, and they quickly become obstacles to joy, peace, and our ability to cope with problems. As an illness progresses, worries intensify, especially when we feel we are not in control of what is happening. How can we break this cycle?

Difficult thoughts came to me again and again as I lay on my back looking out over the Kwilu River—especially the thought that I could do nothing about my back. One day, God impressed a simple question on my heart: *Whose back is this?* Of course it is my back, mine to use. But God made it and God is in control of it and wants to be in control of me. My worrying about what happened would be of no earthly good to my back; in fact, it would impede my recovery. So I released my back to God.

The prayer of release is a powerful prayer. I say to God: "You are in charge. Tell me what, if anything, you want me to do. But I am giving this situation into your hands to accomplish what I believe is a good plan, even though at the moment I do not understand it."

Release not only frees my mind, it stops my brain from producing neurochemicals that weaken my immune system and impede my recovery powers. No longer do I try to cajole God into doing what I thought was necessary. He made my back; he knows how to fix it.

God did indeed tell me what to do. He gave me orders through my consulting physician:

1. No sitting for a month. I could stand and I could lie down, but I was not allowed to sit. So for a month I had to eat standing up.

2. Regular exercise. I was to swim, bicycle, and do back-arching exercises to build up my muscles.

3. I had to learn body mechanics so that I could lift loads, push trucks stuck in the mud, and do whatever else was required *in the proper way.*

4. I had to keep my weight under control. I could put no more load on my back than was absolutely necessary.

The triangle of the healing process was in operation. I had my work to do. My physician gave me further instructions. And God was in charge. He has always had a plan for my life. I have often interfered with it, and perhaps he was using this ruptured disk to give me the time to come to him and return to that plan.

I have found it helpful to write down a list of my worries. This brings problems up into the conscious mind where I can deal with them—problems concerning family, work, conflicting priorities, or whatever. I often seek help from Miriam or from others in resolving these worries. Their wisdom, encouragement, and prayer are invaluable. I take many of them to God, for, as the apostle Peter says, "Dump all your cares [worries] on the Lord because he cares for you" (1 Peter 5:7, my translation).

It is important to deal with worries one at a time and work each one through. The problem causing the worry may not be resolved. Nevertheless, when I share the problem with others and know they are working on it with me, I draw on their strength as well as my own. When I share it with God and have the assurance that he is dealing with the problem with me, I am released, not from working on the problem but from worrying about it. This frees my mind from distress and stops the production of neurochemicals that can weaken my body.

Accept responsibility and deal with guilt

When we are ill, we must ask ourselves some tough but very important questions: Is it possible that, in one way or another I am responsible, at least in part, for my illness? What's more, am I putting obstacles in the way of my recovery?

When I had hepatitis B, I had to ask myself these questions. I did not feel I was responsible for getting the disease; it came in the course of my service as a surgeon. But I certainly was compounding the illness by my overwork and my inadequate handling of stress. I was controlling my own life rather than obeying God's laws and letting him control me. I had to face up to that and correct it.

We walk a fine line when we ask such questions of responsibility. We can go too far in one direction and become obsessed with guilt, real or imagined. This adds unhealthy remorse to an already overburdened immune system. In the other direction, however, is the stubborn rejection of all responsibility and the refusal to deal with real problems that need correction. Sometimes it's a good idea to involve another person as we explore our own part in the situation. We can easily be too hard on ourselves and take on guilt that God would not give us. We can also be completely blind to our own lack of judgment. The wonderful news is that God forgives us when we are in fact guilty. God is in the forgiving business; he enjoys freeing us in this way. All we have to do to receive forgiveness from God is to ask for it.

Spiritual Resources

Prayer

Many articles have appeared in the medical literature describing studies on the effects of prayer on health and healing. Most evidence shows that prayer does favorably influence healing and our recuperative powers.

We can acknowledge that, yes, much of prayer is psychological, or "suggestion," as some would call it. And some of prayer's results may have to do with the power of suggestion. Yet some studies show that sick persons who have been prayed for without their knowledge improve faster than those for whom no prayer has been offered. These studies indicate that there is power in prayer beyond the human psyche. Prayer is tapping into the real power of God and asking God to intervene in our lives.[3]

How shall we pray? When we come to God with our needs, we should be specific, talk with God about our particular problems, and ask for specific help. During my illness with hepatitis B, I prayed for my liver and for the liver cells. I prayed for my appetite and for my physical stamina. I counsel persons who have AIDS to pray for their white blood cells. They can ask God to reinforce the ones they have and to give them more. I suggest that they ask Christ to let his healing power circulate through the blood stream to ferret out viruses, to repair damaged tissues, and to rebuild nerves, glands, connective tissue, or whatever else needs attention. When I pray for a sick person, I bring his or her specific problem to God and ask for help.

If you have arthritis, pray for the lining of your joints. If you have a skin problem, pray for your skin, the blood vessels that go to the affected area, and the connective tissue that is disrupted. If you have frequent infections, pray for your immune system. If the problem is cancer, pray for your "killer cells," those special white blood cells that identify and destroy cells in our body that have become abnormal. Ask God to help them do their work.

We can pray also for our caregivers. They need God's power as they try to help us. We can ask God to direct the thoughts, the analytical skills, and the technical expertise of physicians, nurses, counselors, and all who are trying to help us. We can ask God to guide them to "cover all the bases," to find out all that needs to be done and how best to do it.[4]

The wife of a nearby African-American pastor became critically ill with a rare form of pneumonia. She was admitted to the acute care service of the hospital and put under deep sedation. The hope was that by reducing her bodily functions to a minimum, her recuperative powers would eventually be able to handle the infection. Two physicians, both Christian, were responsible for her care. They explained to the pastor that his wife would need to be maintained in this condition for up to a month, and that recovery, if it did occur, would require at least six months. They then prayed together, and the physicians asked God to let his power strengthen the immune system of this woman and restore her to health. Each day as they came by on rounds, they prayed for her with the pastor and the family.

The caregivers were amazed when, after five days, most of the signs of infection had disappeared. They stopped the heavy sedation, and after two more days in intensive care, they moved her to a private room. Within a week she was discharged, and after three more weeks she had resumed normal activities. The fervent prayer of those who live in a close relationship with God can act as a pathway for God to work in effective ways.

The Lord's Supper

If you have a personal relationship with Jesus Christ, you have available to you a ceremony or sacrament that has great symbolic power. It is the Lord's Supper, or the Eucharist as many call it. It symbolizes what Christ has done for us through his life, death, and resurrection. He has saved us from sin and eternal separation from God; he has healed us and has cleansed our lives, and he has reconciled us to God. Unfortunately, in many churches the Lord's Supper has become simply a routine. We rush through it at the end of the Sunday worship, glancing at our watches in our hurry to finish and go on our way. How tragic this is, for we fail completely to honor the Lord with our praise and to avail ourselves of what he has done for us.

The bread, in whatever form it may be—leavened

or unleavened, wafer, loaf, or biscuit—is the symbol of Christ's body. When I partake of the bread, I say to Christ that I am taking into my whole being his life-giving power, and I thank him for making this available to me. My heart hears this and remembers again that Christ's power is within my body, soul, and spirit. His power can give me strength, can help me cope with the problems I face, and can reinforce my body's systems and functions.

When I take the cup—wine or juice—I am drinking the symbol of Christ's blood, which he gave voluntarily for me. I am taking into my whole being his power to forgive my sins, to heal the wounds of my heart, to repair the brokenness of my spirit, and to renew the strength of my body. During the times I have struggled with illness, the Lord's Supper has been of great help to me in lifting me into his presence and in making my heart more aware of his presence and power within me. On occasion it was in the quietness of my room, administered by a servant of the Lord. During periods of health and active service, participation in the Lord's Supper with others renews my joy, my fellowship with the Lord, and the strength of my whole life.

When I am having a problem in my heart, I confess this to God first. Then I drink the symbol of Christ's blood and ask him to cleanse my heart of all that is sinful, impure, and inconsistent. Inner peace and joy return, and they strengthen my body. The Lord's Supper can have great healing power if we enter into it with our mind, soul, and spirit.

The healing Presence

King David said, "You will show me the path of life; in your presence is fullness of joy. At your right hand are pleasures forevermore" (Psalm 16:11, NKJV).

There is real healing power in our awareness of the presence of the Almighty God. That awareness brings a sense that somehow all things fit together, although I may not understand how. It assures me that Someone greater than me is in charge, Someone who loves me, and Someone who is altogether trustworthy. When my heart understands that I am in the hands of the Almighty, this brings peace to the center of my being. From there, this peace can permeate my whole self.

At times when I call on God, nothing happens. Where is he when I need him? A gentle reminder comes: "I am always with you. Where can you go where I am not present?" I then realize that the problem is not with God; it is in my inability to sense his presence. Even when I sense nothing, God is with me. When my mind can understand that, God's power can heal me.

The parables of Jesus are cryptic stories with many dimensions. We are familiar with Jesus' parable about the Good Samaritan (Luke 10:25-37). We understand from this story that our neighbor is anyone, anywhere, who is in need and that God wants us to help them. Let's look at another dimension of this story.

I have often felt that I am that "certain man" who is wounded and lying beside the road. Who among us has never been wounded? Who among us has never been in need of help? As I lie there hurting and desperately waiting for help, my religious self comes by, my church-going, tithe-giving, and rules-abiding self. I seek for healing from my religion, but I do not find it. Religious activities as such have little healing power. Next comes my intellectual self. I reason about my wounds. I analyze them, try to determine the causes and what I can do, and search within myself for ways to assuage my pain and find healing. But my intellectual self cannot heal me.

When I have come to the end of my own resources and recognize that I need help, a Stranger approaches on a donkey. At first I may not recognize him, for he seems to be of a different color, or to speak a different language—somehow, he is strange. But when he stops, gets off his donkey, pours oil and wine on my wounds, and bandages them, I recognize him as Jesus, the Christ, the Lord of life and our Healer. Then he takes me to where others can care for me until full healing comes. It is the presence of this Stranger, the Lord Christ, who brings healing to my deep wounds.

It is possible to bring a loved one into the healing presence of God through prayer. We can do this even from a distance of thousands of miles. Joel was the fourth child of a missionary family in Africa. When he was four months old, a missionary nurse noted with alarm that Joel's head was too big. Two pediatricians were nearby, and they confirmed her suspicions: Joel was rapidly developing hydrocephalus, excess liquid in the head due to a blockage of spinal fluid.

Three days later Joel arrived in Toronto with his mother, and the following day, Sunday, he was admitted to a children's hospital. The physicians confirmed the clinical diagnosis made a few days earlier.

That same day, six thousand miles away in Kinshasa, thirty of us gathered together to pray for Joel. I was asked to be in charge of this gathering. An initial time of fellowship and worship created a spirit of oneness among us. Joel's father then described what he knew of the problem, and we began to pray. We prayed for Joel, for his mother, for the caregivers in Toronto, and we asked God to heal the fluid blockage in Joel's head.

After we had prayed for some minutes, I suggested that each of us picture in our mind Jesus standing in the middle of our circle. Then I said, "Let us now put

Joel in Jesus' hands so that he can hold him. In the presence of Jesus there is great healing power." We truly sensed the presence of the Lord Christ in our midst, sang the doxology, and went home.

The following morning, in Toronto, a spinal tap revealed a tinge of blood in Joel's spinal fluid. A radio-opaque dye was injected, and the doctors watched it flow unimpeded into the ventricles of the brain and then return freely to the spinal canal. The next morning the physicians informed Joel's mother that, although Joel had indeed had a blockage of the fluid, it had somehow ruptured and all was now clear. The presence of blood in the spinal fluid indicated that the rupture had just occurred, perhaps on Sunday. In our prayer in central Africa we put Joel in Jesus' hands. About that time, in Toronto, the blockage ruptured. Were those two events related? I believe so.

The presence of the Stranger, the Lord Christ, has great healing power. He asks us to work together to bring our wounded selves before him so that he might heal us body and soul.

Get the help you need

When we are ill, most of us need help. We can do only so much on our own. We need the help of diagnostic skills, medicines, and technical interventions of one sort or another. We need the help of compassionate caregivers as we walk through the often difficult or painful days, months, or even years of the illness. Illness saps not only our physical strength but also our emotional and spiritual energies. Many times we find we cannot muster either the will or the psychic energy to deal in depth with what we have been talking about here. We need help, and that is why a team of people working together is so important. Family, friends, a community of faith, and caregivers of many kinds—

this is the team that can bring together the many things we need to help us on the journey toward wholeness.

In the final analysis, however, what is crucial is our own response to the disease, disaster, or accident. Do we regard it as a tragedy or a challenge? If we accept it as a challenge, we choose the way of hope. Our caregivers can then reinforce that hope, and our hope can encourage them. Yet some tough issues remain, and we now turn to them.

12

Finding Hope in Dark Places

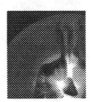

In spite of all the therapeutic resources available to us from our technology and our faith, we are still left with many difficult situations that require much wisdom, patience, and courage. Most of us, at one time or another, will need to walk through dark places, even the valley of the shadow of death. These dark places take many forms: incurable disease, protracted and debilitating illness, permanent disfigurement or malformation, and, ultimately, death of people close to us.

In times of great difficulty what we seek most is hope. By its very nature bad news tends to destroy hope. And once hope is destroyed, despair sets in with all of its depressing effects. Not only do we struggle in our outward, daily life under the burden of despair, but our inner life—immune system, emotions, spirit—is weakened. The only way to battle this all-consuming despair is to renew our hope. But where do we find it?

Hope and the Truth

It may seem strange, but there is an intimate connection between the truth and genuine hope. Hope based on ignorance, conjectures, or lies will not stand the test of time. To have genuine hope we must know the truth.

In our hospital in the Congo, when I have to present bad news to a sick person, I tell a story that helps to make clear the importance of truth. Many years ago a rebellion broke out in the Kwilu region near to us. Young insurgents hid in the forest and launched attacks on government centers. The government did not know who they were, how many of them were involved, or where they were hiding. Because of the government's ignorance, the rebellion spread to many areas and became a threat to the entire country.

The government got smart. They sent out informants to find out what was going on. They gathered extensive information. When the government finally knew the true situation, it was able to carry on an effective campaign to stamp out the rebellion and save the country. In other words, a knowledge of the truth enabled the government to cope with the problem and handle it properly.

A serious illness can be compared to a rebellion going on inside the sick person. The rebels may be bacteria, viruses, cancer cells, or something else. As we have seen, we have built-in defenses against these invaders. However, our natural defenses often need the help of modern medicine, of expert counseling and care, and of the resources of our faith. In order to make that possible, we do extensive tests to gather all possible information about the nature of the illness.

When the information I've gathered about a sick person indicates that there is indeed bad news, I explain as much of the situation as I think he or she can understand. At the same time I emphasize the good news that coping mechanisms are available and that we will use them together. I discovered a long time ago that the *truth plus hope* make a very beneficial combination.

I also realized that the truth cannot be hidden. Something deep within a person's spirit senses the outlines of reality. Somehow our intuition informs us that something serious is wrong. If the details of that reality are not made clear, however, confusion reigns and leads to fear. So a knowledge of the truth, *given at the right time and in the right way*, removes the confusion and fear. The truth, even though it may be difficult, restores the peace of mind that can indeed strengthen the immune system and the recovery process, even when recovery seems unlikely.

Facing Fear

Bad news does bring fear, and fear can depress us and impair our immune system. But fear can be dispelled when we understand what is wrong and can then determine that we will face this difficult reality. Most of us do rise to a challenge. Truth given with hope can help us mobilize our own coping mechanisms and can enable family and caregivers to work more effectively with us.

During my surgical residency many years ago, I cared for a nineteen-year-old soldier who had a malignant melanoma on his face that had spread to lymph nodes in his neck. Since I had established a rapport with him, the chief of service asked me to tell the young man his diagnosis and discuss the options with him. We talked first about his military life and how he had been trained to cope with an enemy. This involves developing a battle plan with various strategies.

I then explained that this brown tumor on his face was a formidable enemy, but one that could be overcome. I outlined the options available: radical surgery on the face and neck, or disfiguring radiation. I helped this young man and his father face the decision. I appealed to the discipline the army had instilled in him and to his own wisdom and courage to face difficult decisions. He accepted his diagnosis, opted for radical surgery, and did beautifully. In his mind, the disfiguring scars on his neck were a small price to pay for restoration to health and long life. The truth plus hope can overcome many obstacles.

So we must not be afraid to face a difficult reality. Fear will not help us. Instead, we must face reality as a challenge and an opportunity to mobilize our own coping mechanisms and those of our family and caregivers.

Hope and a Reason to Live

An essential part of hope is the ability to see a meaning or purpose in life. I have seen persons with cancer or with HIV/AIDS add months and sometimes even years to their lives because they have found a reason to keep on living. For some, the purpose has been to see their children through school. For others it has been to finish fleshing out their own visions and accomplishments.

Reaching forward to attain a goal fixes one's attention toward what lies ahead, and this can stimulate coping mechanisms and mobilize physical resources for combating the destructive effects of disease.

Finding a Purpose in the Illness

Why am I ill? Why did this happen to me? It's perfectly reasonable and legitimate to search for a purpose in your illness. Such a search can even be therapeutic. Jesus himself recognized how important this was. In John chapter 9 we read about Jesus and his disciples meeting a blind man sitting by the side of the road. He had been born blind. The disciples asked Jesus why. Had the man sinned, or was he blind because his parents had sinned? John recorded Jesus' reply: "His blindness has nothing to do with his sins or with his parents' sins. He is blind so that God's power might be seen in him" (John 9:3).

Somehow I believe that there was more in that conversation than what John recorded. I suspect the man himself entered into the discussion, for surely he had many questions. The point is that Jesus considered the question "Why was this man born blind?" important enough to deal with it before he actually healed the man. Jesus responded to the man's intellectual problem prior to healing his physical problem. Jesus assured the man that his blindness had a purpose, a purpose now about to be fulfilled.

A disease, disaster, or accident may indeed seem senseless. Nevertheless, can we give it a meaning? Can we find a purpose in it and make it do something good for us? I think we can start by asking these questions:

- What lessons can I learn from the illness?
- Does the illness seem to indicate certain changes I should make in my life?
- Do I need to listen more to my wife (or husband) and to my children? Do I need to spend more time with them?

- How willing am I to show other people kindness and to help them instead of just seeing how they can help me?
- What am I doing with my life? Where am I headed?
- Where is God in this illness? Is he trying to tell me something?

As we consider these questions, a wise helper, family member, friend, pastor, or physician can be of great assistance. As a physician, I cannot tell you the meaning of your illness. But I can dialogue with you as you seek to discover it for yourself.

When I had hepatitis B, God was working in my life. Did God make me sick? I don't know, and I refuse to second-guess God. What I do know is that *when I asked God questions about my hepatitis, he gave me answers about my life.* My hepatitis became for me a symbol that something in my lifestyle needed correcting. When I went to God, he helped me understand that my workaholic lifestyle was bad for my health. In fact, it was killing me.

Whatever the illness may be, it can be an event through which God can speak. No one else can tell you what God may be trying to say to you through the illness. So when an illness or a disaster does come, I would encourage you to go to God, to ply him with questions, and to wrestle with him about the answers. This is how our faith grows, and it is how we gain wisdom.

In a real sense, an illness is an event with a voice. It is a teacher. Seeking healing and recovery is normal and very important. Seeking wisdom is even better. Happy is the person who can say, "I have recovered from my illness, and I am wiser because of it." And she or he can be happy even if it is necessary to say, "I have not recovered from my disease, but I am becoming wiser because of it." The attainment of wisdom is almost always possible even if full recovery is not.

Restoring Relationships

The physical healing of cancer, HIV, or other debilitating diseases may be beyond our grasp, at least for the moment. The healing of relationships, however, is not. The helpful counsel of a wise friend or family member may be of great help in resolving painful relationships. This has great importance when we are in a dark valley.

Gottfried is one of my close colleagues. He knew that his father back in Germany was suffering from cancer. When he received word that his father had only a short time to live, Gottfried returned to Germany to spend time with him.

Gottfried knew that his father had serious problems in his relationships with many people, including Gottfried's mother, the other children, and Gottfried himself. Quietly, and with much prayerful preparation, Gottfried talked to his father about the need for forgiveness of his own sins and the importance of forgiving others and working through years of misunderstandings, resentments, and bitterness. His father was not only able to forgive people who had offended him but was also able to ask for forgiveness from people he had offended. He had sometimes spoken angrily to his wife and hurt her deeply. He asked her forgiveness for that. He also asked his children for forgiveness for the many times that, when they needed him, he was not there. He became reconciled to his wife and to his sons and daughters.

One burden in particular was weighing on his father's heart. A small stream went through the village, and the village authorities had made a rule that no one could fish in that stream. Gottfried's father had broken that rule, eaten some lovely fish, and felt guilty about it. So, as Gottfried was helping his father rebuild relationships with others, Gottfried invited the mayor and his wife to come in for tea. When the father confessed his "sin" to the mayor, the mayor smiled broadly. "My dear friend, I have eaten several fish from that stream myself. I will forgive you if you will forgive me."

When the end of his earthly journey came a short time later, Gottfried's father passed into eternity at peace. His family and friends, although grieving, were also at peace. If we can bring peace into our relationships, that peace can help us cope with even the darkest of circumstances.

The Bible is full of help in the area of relationships. God is the great Healer of all relationships, and he can help us work through ours. We should strive to be at peace with everyone. Forgiving others and accepting their forgiveness bring peace to the heart and strength to the body. Even with persons who have no desire for reconciliation or who have already departed from this life, forgiveness is possible. The heart can be healed of the anger, rivalries, jealousy, and bitterness of those hurting relationships, and the God of peace can then fill it with his peace.

This is of great importance as we approach our final journey. It is also important for those who will remain behind. Grief is a normal and often intense emotion that follows the departure of a loved one. But if we can restore peace to our relationships before we die, this peace can assuage the grief of those who remain after us. This is a wonderful gift we can give to our loved ones.

Changing What Can Be Changed

What can we do when the cancer continues to spread in spite of the best therapy, or the headaches will not diminish, or the HIV will not go away? Have we failed? Has our faith been insufficient? Is there unconfessed sin, unsolved conflict, or buried anger?

Wanting to be in charge comes naturally to human beings. We want to overcome all obstacles. Reality however is against us. Many things in this life are beyond our control. Among them is the inevitability of physical death. How can we face death when we still want to recover? After having tried everything including prayer, counseling, faith, and all manner of treatments—while the disease continues on its destructive course—what more can we do?

A serious injury or a debilitating disease can shorten life or permanently disfigure the body. It can disturb our sense of worth, our dignity, and our creativity, all of which compose God's image within us. Furthermore, the disease or disability diminishes our physical and perhaps psychological capacities to be creative, to be in control of life, and to contribute to the world. Our place in which to be somebody has shrunk. Is everything beyond control, or are there still things we can change?

Here is the dilemma. As the disease increases, the fear and anxiety increase with it. These feelings depress the immune system and recuperative powers, the very things we need to fight the disease. We are caught in a vicious cycle from which no escape seems possible.

Viktor Frankl, who survived inhuman circumstances in a Nazi concentration camp during the Holocaust, says, "Everything can be taken from a man but one thing: the last of the human freedoms—to choose one's attitude to any given set of circumstances, to choose one's own way."[1]

In the face of advancing disease, permanent disability, or approaching death, we still have a choice. We can choose our attitudes toward our circumstances and toward life in general. Recognizing and accepting reality is helpful. Knowing the truth can be therapeutic. Facing and accepting the reality of disease is more healthy than trying to change the unchangeable. When we face reality positively and accept it as a challenge, we sometimes find that what we thought was unchangeable begins to change—because we have changed.

In times of great stress I take pen and paper and make a list of all the problems I am facing. I have found this to be a useful exercise when I deal with serious illness. What do we deal with when we are ill? Pain, weakness, the inability to do this or that, the high cost of treatment, and all of the outward circumstances that press so heavily on us. We can add to that list the dark thoughts, bad dreams, grief, anger, frustration, and anxiety that we want to get rid of but can't. We now have a detailed list of what is involved in our struggle.

After I make my problem list, I put it in front of me. I take a red pen and put a check by all of those obstacles and negative factors that cannot be changed. I take a blue pen and put a check by those factors I think I can change. This includes my feelings and thoughts, for they are factors within myself. On a separate sheet of paper, I rewrite those items marked in blue. This is my "controllable list."

In chapter 11 we looked at the many ways we can cope with serious illness. I have used them all and found them helpful. What is especially helpful is the knowledge that I am doing something, and that I am in charge of at least a little bit of my life. This sends a message to my recuperative powers: "Let's keep going; one tiny step at a time."

It can be especially helpful to focus on other people. So many times when I have called a sick friend to give encouragement and comfort, that encouragement has come back to me. Praying for others or for particular projects, even when we are seriously ill, takes our thoughts away from our troubles and gets us involved in things beyond ourselves. During these moments our immune system is free from the stressful chemicals our worried thoughts produce.

Even in the dark valley we can change our atmosphere. We can surround ourselves with good things: music, flowers, helpful books, pictures of beautiful scenes. This can let the spirit move upward, and we can then thank God for all that is good. Praise to God gives hope and can strengthen our recuperative powers and our will to live.

The prophet Jeremiah suffered throughout his life. Yet he did not lose hope. "The thought of my pain and my destitution is like bitter poison. I think of it constantly, and my spirit is depressed. Yet hope returns when I remember this one thing: the steadfast love of the Lord never ceases, his mercies never come to an end; they are new every morning; great is his faithfulness. The Lord is all I have, and so in him I put my hope" (Lamentations 3:19-24, my paraphrase).

In the face of overwhelming disease, we still have a choice, the choice of our attitude toward life. I can choose to accept myself; I can choose to accept God; and I can choose to accept the declaration that God, as a loving Father, is working in my life to bring it to fullness and to restore his image in me. This restoration is taking place now and will be completed in eternity. In so choosing, I find peace, and that peace can change my life, heal my spirit, and it may strengthen my body.

Where Is God When I Need Him?

Is God really present in the valley of the shadow of death? Is God present only when I feel that he is with me? Or is he present no matter what I feel?

In the book of Isaiah, God gives a marvelous promise to his people. "Do not be afraid—I will save you. I have called you by name—you are mine. When you pass through deep waters, I will be with you; your troubles will not overwhelm you. When you pass through the fire, you will not be burned; the hard trials that come will not hurt you. For I am the Lord your God" (Isaiah 43:1-3).

Five deep truths stand out in this promise:

1. *When we come into a relationship with God, he knows our name.* We belong to him and have a place in his family. He cares for us.

2. *Difficulties will come. The waters of trouble can be deep.* The fires of adversity will burn. God has never promised us immunity from difficulties. They are a part of life for each of us.

3. *Nevertheless, in every difficulty, God is with us.* He accompanies us and goes with us through the deep water, through the fire, and through whatever the difficulty may be, even terminal illness.

4. *We will get to the other side because God is with us.* We may not find strength or courage on our own, but we can draw on God's strength. His

presence shall never depart from us no matter how we feel, and we can safely trust in him even though we do not understand the situation, see its conclusion, or know if that conclusion is in this world or in the next.

5. *God says, "When you pass through the fire, you will not be burned."* In other words, your true being will not be destroyed because God is the God of life. The physical body will perish, now or later, but not your real self. This is why the Bible speaks about the "living hope" (1 Peter 1:3). This living hope means an eternal relationship with God, and it comes to us when we enter into a relationship with Jesus Christ. This hope is available to every one of us no matter what our outward circumstances or condition may be. According to the Bible, this hope includes the renewal in eternity of our physical body with flesh and bones that will never die.

In this passage from Isaiah we see the reality of suffering from God's point of view. Suffering is real and it is a part of our lives. God has willed it to be so because he has a purpose in it. And he is with us in it even if we are unaware of his presence. We can count on that.

Suffering is tough. We don't want it, and when it comes, we want to get rid of it as quickly as possible. Yet often we cannot escape it. Isaiah assures us, however, that even in the deepest suffering, we do not need to be alone. If we reach out to God, he will reach out to us and will be with us.

At the core of our being is the deep longing or desire to live in relationship with God. God is our Creator, one who loves us eternally and who gives ultimate meaning and purpose to life. Our heart senses this longing, and in the depths of our heart we are lonely without God.

We also long to understand the whys and wherefores of our suffering, but this is not always possible. In that case the knowledge of God's presence can be of great comfort. King Solomon wrote, "Trust in the Lord with all your heart. Never rely on what you think you know. Remember the Lord in everything you do, and he will show you the right way" (Proverbs 3:5-6).

Have you satisfied that desire by allowing God to fill the center of your being? This is the most fundamental change you can make in this life, and it can be made even when all other changes seem impossible. If God is indeed already dwelling in your heart, you can invite him into the deepest recesses of your being. Open the doors into all the rooms of your heart and submit to God your deepest longings and desires. His peace can then fill you completely and heal your spirit—the real *you* he created in the beginning.

Looking Squarely at Death

Death will come to all of us. It does us no good to deny that reality; in fact, such a negative approach can be harmful to us and to the people we love. The mature approach to dying and death is to face reality and make adequate preparations for it. How do we prepare to die?

In 1959, several months prior to our departure for what was then the Belgian Congo, Miriam and I began our preparations in earnest. We each had to have a passport. In addition to having many things to pack, we had to be sure we were leaving our affairs in good order. Failure in this would unnecessarily burden our family, who would remain at home.

Similar to a departure into a new country is our final departure into a new life. I do not think of my death as loss. Instead, I think of it as a journey, as moving into a new home and a new place of service. However, for such a journey, I need a "passport." Jesus said, "I am the way, the truth, and the life; no one goes to the Father except by me" (John 14:6). The presence of Christ in my heart is my passport with a permanent resident visa stamped into it. With this passport in hand, I have no fear when finally I approach the "immigration authorities" of eternity.

I also need to make sure my affairs are in order. Financial matters, wills, property, and personal belongings—I must handle these before I leave. I must handle them clearly and correctly to prevent the painful tensions that would arise among family members if I left my personal affairs in disorder.

I truly believe that God is the God of life, not of death. Yet as death looms large, our hearts need solace as well as courage. The deeply disturbing question of why can be very unsettling. If God is the God of life, why must we die?

Why Do Sparrows Fall?

Jesus once said, "For only a penny you can buy two sparrows, yet not one sparrow falls to the ground without your Father's consent" (Matthew 10:29). Here is a difficult question. If God is good and if he loves sparrows, why do they fall?

Job wrestled with this question. He had lost almost everything of value in his life. He was seriously ill with what seemed to him like a hopeless disease. He turned to his friends for wisdom and solace but did not find it. He turned to God to argue with him, even to express his deep anger and bitterness toward him, but God didn't supply simple answers. Job sought life and found only darkness and pain.

What Job did not understand, nor could he in the midst of his illness, was that all of these difficulties had a meaning and purpose. His faith was being tested. God knew Job and knew the depth of his faith. God was willing to allow Job to suffer to the very depths of his being as a witness to the people of his own world and to the spiritual powers of darkness that the faith of a person could endure even the deepest of trials.

Job did not know what God was up to, nor can we fully understand what God is up to in our lives. However, Job asked God, and God finally answered him. Job argued with God, and God honored him by meeting with him. We too can ask, wrestle, and argue with God, provided we are willing to listen to the answers God gives. Job did not die of his illness, but many people do, and all of us will eventually die. Where is God in this? Why is physical death part of his plan for all of us? Why do the sparrows he has made fall? Consider these stories.

When a son goes away

I stood at Patrice's bedside with his mother and father, two of the bravest people I know. They had cared for their son constantly for more than a year, at home and through many long days and nights at the hospital. A few minutes before, Patrice had told them goodbye and then quietly slipped away.

When Patrice first came to our hospital, he was seriously ill. He was a thirty-four-year-old unmarried mechanic who had lived in the city of Kinshasa for many years, and his way of life had exposed him to HIV. When he arrived at Vanga, he was emaciated and was suffering from severe diarrhea, mouth sores, and bloody urine. We gave him many antibiotics, but there was little improvement.

Mrs. Matala and some on the nursing staff spent hours with Patrice, talking, counseling, and praying. Patrice opened his heart to Christ and he found a new life and a reason to live. His appetite returned, his diarrhea and bloody urine stopped, and flesh came back on his bones. After three months, he left the hospital and went to live with his parents in a nearby village. We would see him make regular visits to the hospital; he'd bring his guitar and sing and talk with both patients and staff. Often he came to the Bible studies and to the Sunday morning worship service at the hospital.

After a few months of illness-free living, Patrice went back to Kinshasa to be with his friends. Three months later he returned, once again seriously ill. This time it was clear that the years of infection had exhausted his immune system and that another remission was unlikely. His spirit, however, was undaunted, and he remained at peace until the end, singing, talking with others, and encouraging the staff.

As we stood by the bedside, I put my arm around his father's shoulders and said to both parents, "Patrice has now been fully healed. The enemy of our souls, the devil, determined to destroy your son, but God healed his heart, soul, and spirit, and has prepared a new body for him. All that remains for the devil is this mortal body, and it soon will be gone." Through their tears, they nodded assent and smiled, for they knew they would once again be united. This was the moment of closure. A "sparrow" had fallen, but had Patrice really "fallen"?

It is a heavy task to walk alongside persons who have AIDS. We know there is no cure. Yet we know there is healing for heart, soul, and spirit, and that this healing leads to life. We find great encouragement in knowing that most of the HIV patients we've had the privilege of accompanying on their journey have found that healing and new life. We lose the AIDS battle, but the greater victory has already been won.

When a child goes away

To me, the name Robert Mindana means heaven. It has been almost thirty years since Robert went there, but I can still see his bright smile and sharp eyes. Although he was sixteen years old, he had the stature of a ten-year-old. He had been born with a serious malformation of the heart, and this had retarded his physical growth. Since this was in the bush of central Africa, with no diagnostic means available other than eyes, ears, and a tired old military X-ray machine, we could not determine the exact nature of Robert's malformation. Even if that had been possible, we couldn't have done anything about it.

Robert's father was a village pastor, and during Robert's cardiac crises he would bring him in to the hospital at Vanga. We kept him on digoxin and treated his crises with the usual remedies for heart failure. In the intervals between crises, Robert would attend school, for he was an intelligent boy.

Late one evening, when Robert had been in the hospital almost a month with his latest crisis, his father came to tell me that Robert had just died. Through his tears, he told me his son's final words. His father was at the bedside when Robert called him to sit on the bed with him.

"Papa," he said, "I see Jesus and he is calling me to come to him. I love you and Mama. I have nothing in my heart against anyone. I am at peace and I am now going to live with Jesus." He then embraced his father, lay back on his pillow, closed his eyes, and left.

We could say that Robert Mindana had fallen. But is that really the right verb to use?

When a baby dies

Why do babies die? We don't know, and so confusion, frustration, and even anger are added to our grief. "God, why did you give us this little one and then take him away from us?" This question has often come into my heart as I have looked at a perfectly formed baby lying lifeless on the delivery table. I may know the medical cause of death, but the purpose of the death evades me. How can we cope when a baby dies?

When our daughter-in-law Jackie was five months pregnant with their fourth child, a routine ultrasound examination showed that something was wrong. There was no amniotic fluid around the baby. A second, more extensive examination confirmed the doctors' suspicions: the little one had no kidneys. The kidneys produce urine, and the amniotic fluid, which protects the developing baby, is made up mostly of the baby's urine. Within the uterus, the baby can grow and develop without kidneys, but once outside the uterus, the baby can live only a few hours if at all. Since there was no hope for life after birth, the medical team suggested that the pregnancy be terminated if Paul and Jackie so wished. There was no danger to Jackie, however, if the pregnancy continued until term.

Jackie and Paul did three things. They talked to God about this. Their primary question to the Lord was not why. Rather it was, What do you wish us to do with this new life you have entrusted to us? They knew they were responsible and accountable for this new person and that their primary accountability was to God himself, who had given this little one to them. So they went to him for wisdom.

They also talked to their three children, who were

eagerly anticipating the arrival of a new sister or brother. Carefully Paul and Jackie explained that their new baby was sick and probably would not be able to live with them. Joshua, age six, insisted on knowing why God would give them a new brother or sister who could not live with them. He also asked that, if the baby did go straight to heaven, could God give them another brother or sister? Steven, age four, wondered how the little one would grow up. Christy, at two, kept on smiling and pursuing her happy ways only vaguely aware of the drama taking place within her mother's tummy.

Then Jackie and Paul went to their family and to their wide circle of Christian brothers and sisters on three continents. Immediately they were surrounded by praying people who also encouraged their faith in a loving God. Although they were in England and we were in the United States, we walked this journey with them through daily contacts by e-mail and telephone.

Jackie and Paul know that God is the author of life and the creator of each one of us. They know also that life is forever, not in this world, but in eternity. They believed God had a plan for this little life even though they did not fully understand it. So they made the decision to leave their little one entirely in the hands of God, allowing the pregnancy to continue to term. We cannot know God's thoughts nor his timing, but we can affirm them even without understanding the course of events. With this decision made, Jackie and Paul found peace.

They likewise decided that they would pour as much love as could possibly be poured into a little one in utero. This is no time to deny reality but to accept what has come and to make every effort to fulfill the roles of a loving mother and father. They wanted to name the baby so that they could talk to him or her directly and pray by name. But because there was no amniotic fluid, determination of gender was not possible before birth. However, they believed that God already knew the name. In my own heart, I was at peace praying for our little one, whom I felt would be our grandson.

Jackie and Paul were determined that, when the birth occurred, for however many minutes or hours of earthly life was granted to him or her, they would surround the little one with loving arms and prayer. Then when the moment of departure came, they would transfer the infant confidently into the loving arms of Jesus. They believed firmly that God's plan for their little one was the best plan and so they placed this little life entirely in God's hands. They believed God was accomplishing his eternal purpose for their child, and they refused to interfere in this. They also knew God was helping their own faith to grow. They went through sadness, grief, and the pain of loss and separation. Yet underneath all of that was the unshakable belief that God knows what he is doing, and that what he does with us and for us is to remake us more and more in his image. After all, he gave his Son for us.

One warm summer afternoon in Michigan soon after we learned of the problem of our new grandchild, I was picking blueberries with two of our other grandchildren. As the berries went plunk, plunk, plunk into our tins, my thoughts wandered upward.

"Lord, who will teach our little one how to pick blueberries, which ones are ripe and which ones are not? How can he know the sheer delight of the sight and taste of ripe berries, where to find the choicest blackberries, or how to recognize trillium or lilies of the valley in the spring? The taste of freshly roasted peanuts, and the delicate scent of roses—will he ever experience these joys? Jesus, will you have time to show him all these wonders of your creation, teaching him all he needs to know?"

These were the questions of my heart. They were not complaints or accusations. I just wanted to know. Jesus gently replied in the depths of my spirit.

"Is not your own mother here with me now? She knows trillium, lilies of the valley, and all about blueberries. Your father, this little one's great-grandfather, knew where to find the best blackberries and he has already found them here. He will be overjoyed to pick the finest blackberries with his dearly beloved great-grandchild.

"There are many other teachers here besides me. Moses is here, Ruth and Mary, Peter and John, George MacDonald, C. S. Lewis, and George Washington Carver. George knows almost as much about flowers and peanuts as I do, because I taught him.

"You may be sure that when this little child comes here, I will be the first to take his hand. I will introduce him to his great-grandparents and to the host of teachers and companions he will have. You may be sure he will learn much and will experience the sights, sounds, tastes, and odors of the beauties of heaven beside which those of earth are only a dim shadow. When you arrive, and when this little one's own mother and father arrive, you will meet your lovely, strong, spiritually mature child and grandchild who will then be your teacher." The berries in my tin were wet with my tears, but the grief in my heart was mingled with the calm assurance that our loving Father will care for this little one even better than could his own earthly mother and father, good as they are.

In the early morning hours of Sunday, October 12, 1997, little Michael was born. He lay quietly in his mother's arms as his father talked to him and prayed with him. In God's marvelous wisdom and goodness, he allowed me to participate in this birth. It occurred during a three-day stopover in England as I was returning from Africa to the United States. So I also had the wonderful privilege of holding this precious boy in my arms and talking to him. Jackie's mother brought Joshua, Steven, and Christy in to see their little brother so they could hold him in their memory. When, after the space of about twenty minutes, his earthly life was finished, we committed our little Michael into the loving care of Jesus who had already prepared a place for him. Jackie and Paul now have four children in their family; three are with them, and one is with Jesus.

A small stone in the cemetery in Accrington, Lancashire, England marks the short earthly life of Michael Fountain, much loved, and who is now with the Father who is love. In my own heart I can envisage the reunion of Paul and Jackie with Michael. I can hear Michael saying to his parents, "Thank you. You loved me, cared for me, and allowed me to live with you as long as possible, and you committed me into the hands of Jesus. Let me now teach you what I have learned so far in God's presence."

Michael has taught us a precious lesson. Heaven is now so much more real because one of our own children is there waiting for us.

Why does God create a new person who cannot live in this life? Why are there miscarriages, stillborn babies, and infant deaths? We cannot know for sure. However, could it be that God wants special people in eternity, people who are fully human but in whom his image has never been defaced by sin and rebellion?

Which brings us back to our burning question: why do sparrows fall? To me the answer has become clear: so they can fly higher.

Death, the Entrance to New Life

Death does not need to mean failure. On the contrary, death can be the realization of ultimate and complete healing. If my mind, heart, and spirit have been healed, physical death then means entrance into a new life. It means being clothed in a new body, one that will permit an eternity of life, of learning, and of service. "Where, Death, is your victory? Where, Death, is your power to hurt? . . . Thanks be to God who gives the victory through our Lord Jesus Christ" (1 Corinthians 15:55, 57).

Appendix:
The Healing Team

Here I want to address my fellow healers: physicians, nurses, psychologists, psychiatrists, and counselors. I include pastors, priests, and concerned family members in these remarks as well, for by listening to sick persons, encouraging them, and caring for them, you also are healers.

When I talk to my doctor colleagues about this approach and how to care for the whole person, the usual response is, "I don't have time to do this." This is absolutely true. As I helped to develop and administer a four-hundred-bed hospital in the Congo and saw multitudes of sick persons, I did not have time for it either. But God showed our hospital how to do it by making it a team approach. We hired Mrs. Matala who, as we have seen, is a trained pastoral caregiver. She is on the hospital staff. Her consulting room is in proximity to the doctors. We refer sick persons to her, and the results have been remarkable. She is a healer just as we physicians are healers.

We call this a pastoral care service. Mrs. Matala and her staff are pastors, caring for the psychological and spiritual needs of sick persons while we health professionals care for their physical needs. Mrs. Matala is an advocate, promoting good health and what is necessary to recover good health. In the same way, we health professionals are advocates for others' healing and health. Medical care and pastoral care thus fit together.

We do not call this a "counseling" service. The terms "counselor" and "counseling" imply that we have the power to tell others how to solve their problems and that we have the authority to "counsel" them as to how they should live. We have neither. We cannot solve another person's problems because we can never fully enter into their situation to identify their problems. If we try to present solutions to them, they are our solutions, not theirs. Only as they find their own solutions and take responsibility for applying them will they take ownership of them. Our role is simply to help them do that. In addition, we do not have the right to tell them how they should live, for that would be an unacceptable imposition.

The French have a wonderful way of expressing this. They call it *la relation d'aide,*—the helping relationship. This emphasizes first of all that we are helpers, not counselors, and that our role is to help sick persons find healing and move toward wholeness. Secondly, it underscores the importance of the relationship between the sick person and the one helping.

The New Testament speaks of the Holy Spirit as the "Paraklete," which means the "one who walks alongside of us to help us, who accompanies us on our journey." All of us on the healing team should see ourselves as those who walk alongside sick persons to help them and to accompany them on their journey toward wholeness.

The Team Approach to Healing

Healing involves the whole person. Physical healing occurs when the anatomy and physiology of the body are restored to functional effectiveness. Health professionals are specially trained for this dimension of healing but need to realize that it occurs more rapidly and completely if other team members are caring for the psychological, social, and spiritual dynamics of the person at the same time. Psychological healing occurs when inner problems of anxiety, conflicts, and painful emotions are resolved. This inner healing facilitates physical healing. Psychology and psychiatry can accomplish much for the healing of the mind and soul.

Healing of the spirit is part of the restoration of the whole person. Christ is the one who heals our spirit by restoring our relationship with God. The presence of the Holy Spirit in the heart of a sick person makes Christ's power available to heal anxiety, disturbing memories, painful emotions, conflicting feelings, and errant desires.

Healing also involves social restoration. Many sick persons have worries and concerns about the cost of health care, about how to obtain other needed services, and about possible changes in living conditions. Social services are an important part of the healing team to help meet these needs. As the social needs are met, worries diminish and the depressive effects of worry and stress are alleviated.

This model works well in a hospital setting. It works equally well on a smaller scale in a clinic or in a private practice setting. What is essential in caring for the whole person is a team of caregivers, large or small, who can care for the full spectrum of the needs of sick persons.

Referral of the Sick Person to the Pastoral Staff

As a physician, I take the initiative in motivating sick persons to participate in pastoral care. In general, members of the health professional staff have the first contact with sick persons. The initial evaluation includes an assessment of their social, psychological, and spiritual needs along with the physical evaluation. This assessment shows if there is a need for pastoral or psychological care, and it serves as a guide in orienting them to the other services they may need.

Referring a sick person to the psychological or pastoral care service requires a careful explanation, for often there is resistance to overcome. Many sick persons believe their illness is a physical problem that requires only a medical or surgical approach to treatment. Any suggestion that emotions or lifestyle may be involved is uncomfortable for them. It implies that they may have to change something in their way of thinking or their behavior, and that they may have to take a responsible part in their healing. Therefore a recommendation that they consult a psychological or pastoral caregiver is threatening to them. This resistance is common; how can we get around it?

After evaluating the physical aspects of the illness, I point out that we are more than just a functioning body. The mind by means of the nervous system rules over the body, gives orders to it, and sets the pace for it. Worries, stress, conflicts, or tensions can diminish the strength and functional effectiveness of the body, making us more susceptible to illness. I often refer to Proverbs 14:30, "Peace of mind makes the body healthy, but envy is like a cancer." Even persons who have no religious faith accept quite readily the statement that our minds influence our bodies and our physical health.

I then explain the importance of dealing with worries, stress, and any other tensions as part of the diagnostic and treatment process. I mention that our staff includes persons skilled in helping those who have worries and emotional concerns. I suggest to the sick person that talking with our pastoral care staff could be of benefit in the treatment process. Relieving worries and concerns, dealing with other problems that might surface, and replacing stress with peace can have positive physical effects that improve the possibilities for healing. Most sick persons recognize the value of this and participate in the pastoral service as their physical evaluation and treatment proceeds.

Dynamics of the Healing Team

Regular communication between members of the healing team is essential. When I refer a sick person to our pastoral care service, I follow up with the staff there. I need to remain aware of how the caring process is proceeding and if social, psychological, or spiritual problems exist that may have physiological effects. I keep the pastoral staff aware of any important changes that occur in a sick person's physical condition or in the treatment schedule. When social concerns are present and the social service staff is involved, they let the medical and pastoral staff know of needs and developments in this area.

As a team we meet together regularly for discussions, problem analysis, prayer, and spiritual encouragement. This helps keep the team spirit alive. It allows for evaluation, trouble shooting, and conflict prevention. Even in the midst of an overcrowded schedule, team meetings are essential. Jesus himself took time not only for private prayer but also to be with his disciples, teaching them and helping them work together. Without such times, the effectiveness of a team rapidly dissipates. Because of this need for regular communication, having the whole team present in one facility is a great advantage.

Prayer strengthens the healing team approach. The members of the team should feel free to pray with each other and as a whole group. Groups of intercessors who provide prayer support for this ministry are of invaluable help. These groups can be in local congregations as well as within the clinic or hospital staff.

Now let's go back to the time constraint problem. My initial evaluation of a sick person, which includes a brief social, psychological, and spiritual evaluation, does take a bit more time than the usual "medical" (physical) consultation. I also spend three to five minutes explaining to the sick person the importance of pastoral care. However, as a result of the pastoral care ministry, far fewer sick persons return to me for followup visits. Prior to this approach, I would become frustrated with the large numbers of persons coming back time after time to say, "Doctor, I have taken all the medicine you gave me, and I still hurt." Because the inner causes of many of their pains are healed by this team approach to caring, many of them have no need to return for further medical help. From this I learned that, in reality, I do not have time *not* to care for the whole person.

Caring—Walking Alongside to Help

All of us on the healing team can have a helping relationship with sick persons. Although the extent to which each of us enters into this relationship will depend on training, skills, and the time available, all of us need to understand what is specifically required of us in order to be good advocates.

The helping relationship

The starting point is to establish a good relationship with the sick person. The initial contact is crucial. Each person I meet with is a unique person of infinite value. I must convey my awareness of that from the first moment. Helping sick persons feel at ease is an art that can be learned. They need the assurance that I am a real person and not just a professional with scientific knowledge. They also need to realize that we are going to work together to find ways that lead toward their healing.

Listening

Listening is a major part of the art of healing. Allow a sick person to tell his or her whole story without interruption. I constantly have to suppress my tendency to interrupt or to change the trend of thought. This can be very damaging to the helping relationship. The time for questions must wait.

Listening is an attitude of openness to the sick person. It involves posture and gestures, for these convey subconscious meaning. How I sit, which way I lean, and the tone of my voice must show that I am open to the one who is suffering. I should convey the sense that I am not only interested but am seeking ways to help.

During the hard winter of 1977–78, I became ill. It was a particularly virulent strain of mycoplasma pneumonia, and I was hospitalized near Chicago. The doctors prescribed intravenous antibiotics, but the infection did not respond. I was afraid, for as a physician I knew what was going on. People die of mycoplasma pneumonia, and I feared I would be among their number. I longed to express my fear, but to whom? The doctors came and went quickly, glancing at their watches as they came by my bed. Friends came, but I could not bare my soul to them. A chaplain stopped by, but he simply gave a word of encouragement and offered a brief prayer. I felt alone. No one would listen.[1]

Each day my wife, Miriam, came and just sat by me. One day I found the courage to pour out to her my anxiety and my fear of dying, and she simply listened. She did not advise me not to be afraid, or rebuke me for lack of faith. After some minutes, she took my hand and read Psalm 91 to me. The final passage burst like the morning sun into the deepest part of my heart: "He shall call upon me, and I will answer him; I will be with him in trouble; I will deliver him, and honor him. With long life will I satisfy him, and show him my salvation" (Psalm 91:15-16, KJV). To my frightened spirit, this was a direct word from God, and I accepted it as a promise from him. My fear departed and my heart was healed. Someone had listened and responded, and God had spoken.[2]

Asking questions

Questions are necessary and as a physician I ask many. Their purpose is to help the sick person describe the illness, and the feelings, concerns, and worries that go with it. Aspects of the illness and especially of the feelings may be difficult to describe. Wise questions can help self-expression and the search for clarity. Many questions will be open ended: "And then what happened?" or "How did that make you feel?" "Can you describe your pain more clearly?" or "In what way are you concerned about that?" These questions should never be threatening, or indicate disapproval or condemnation, for that would effectively shut off the unburdening process.

Discernment

As I listen, I analyze the information I am receiving, not only the spoken information but what I observe. The way a person speaks, nonverbal gestures, and bodily position all help me understand better what is going on and how the sick person feels. For me as a physician and for Mrs. Matala as a pastor, this analysis guides us toward the diagnosis and what seem to be the most appropriate treatment measures to follow.

Sharing experiences

In medical school I was taught that doctors must not share their personal experiences with sick persons. Objectivity, we were told, is important in evaluating a disease process, and to a certain extent this is true. However, illness is more than a disease; it is a disease in a person. I have learned that, when I become subjective to a certain degree, and share something of myself, I make much closer contact with the person. I too have been ill and have gone on the journey toward healing and wholeness, and so I can show that I also am a person with feelings and emotions.

Making recommendations

The time comes when explanations and recommendations are in order. I do not impose instructions or prescribe behavior. Instead, I explain the illness and what we have found so far, giving as much information as I feel the sick person can understand and handle. I describe what we will do to help and what more needs to be done. I then outline a course of action that I believe will be helpful for recovery. I do this in dialogue, not monologue, for questions, discussions, and even objections permit the sick person to participate in the healing process.

Prayer

Prayer is part of this process. In prayer we open our spirit to the leading of the Holy Spirit. While I am with the sick person I often make an instantaneous silent call for guidance, a call for help. If the sick person is open to prayer and asks for it, I will pray audibly, but I never impose prayer on anyone.

Qualifications of an Advocate

Caring for another person is a special calling. It is more a matter of attitude than of actions, of an inner quiet spirit than of outward words and deeds. In theory we health and pastoral professionals have been trained to care for others, but not all of us have learned the attitudes and feelings that are essential for caring. Caring is an art that involves the development of certain skills. What does it require?

Compassion

Compassion means to feel with someone else. We can never feel exactly as another person feels, nor should we try. Nevertheless, we need to communicate our desire to understand what the sick person is feeling.

Affirmation

We affirm a person when we convey the impression that we consider him or her to be someone of real value. I make it a point to learn and remember the name of the sick person before I begin the consultation. Calling a person by name, whether in the clinic, by the bedside, or in the operating room, has a most reassuring effect. It strengthens the helping relationship.

When sick people came to Jesus, he made it a point to affirm them as persons. When the men carrying the paralyzed man interrupted a teaching session of Jesus in Capernaum (Mark 2:1-12), Jesus did not get upset. His first word to the man was, "My son." Rather than scolding him for this rude intrusion into his schedule, he affirmed him, thus gaining his confidence for what was to follow.

Persons with leprosy in Jesus' day were despised, rejected as unclean, and considered as cursed of God. Jesus would have none of that. He touched the man with leprosy who came to him (Mark 1:40-44), a gesture shocking to those who observed it. By so doing, he affirmed him as a person and restored dignity to him.

I recently met Ruth (not her real name), a lovely young woman whom God had redeemed in a remarkable way. She had been born into poverty, drug dealing, and sexual abuse. By the time she entered adolescence, she was a prostitute, a junkie, and a frequent prison inmate. For years her sole motivation was to find sufficient money for her next fix. No one cared for her, and she had no one to care for or to love.

Ruth eventually became pregnant and finally had someone whom she could truly love—her unborn baby. She was then informed that she had HIV and that her baby would probably not live long. During her difficult labor, the doctors and nurses in the hospital were very attentive to the status of her baby while at the same time they totally rejected her as a person. "They said I was just a junkie," Ruth told me. To the doctors' amazement, Ruth finally delivered a fine healthy boy. Then, since she was considered incompetent, they took the baby, the only person she had ever loved, away from her and gave him to someone else.

How can we do this to people? What would Hippocrates say about this? I don't know, but I do know what Jesus would do. He gave his life for this young woman to set her free and to heal her. Jesus knows she bears God's image and has eternal value. With Jesus there are no junkies, prostitutes, or incompetents. There are only people whom he came to seek, to save, and to heal. We are supposed to be like Jesus and to do what he did. Let me add here that this story did not take place in Africa. It occurred in a small city in Pennsylvania.

There is more to this story, however. A prison counselor saw in Ruth something of value. She discerned that God was already working in her heart, and she reached out to her. One day she said to her, "Ruth, I believe in you. Together we are going to work with God's help to restore your life."

Ruth now lives with her three-year-old son and is managing her own business. Her mind, heart, and spirit have been healed, and her body is slowly becoming stronger. Why? Because God in his love spoke to her heart and because another woman, a true advocate, affirmed her and gently poured love into her.

Gentleness

On occasion we have to listen to sordid material. We must listen quietly and accept what we hear without condemnation, judgment, or criticism. We want to get to the bottom of a person's illness. Any reaction of disapproval will cut off further expressions of feelings or behavior and thus keep us from getting the whole picture. A simple nod, or saying, "And then what happened?" is sufficient to enable the person to sense we are listening and we are willing to process whatever comes forth.

Confidentiality

What sick persons reveal to us belongs to them. They are entrusting their story to us because they want our help. However, they are not transferring the ownership of it to us. Absolute confidentiality is essential. Listening and caring are not opportunities for gossip or for acquiring stories to circulate among our friends or family. One reason why so many sick persons have difficulty in talking about their deepest hurts, problems, and fears is the lack of confidence in those to whom they would tell them. As health professionals, pastoral caregivers, and even caring family members or friends, we must keep to ourselves what others entrust to us.

Hope

"A physician can sometimes heal, can often relieve, and can always comfort." This statement is usually ascribed to Hippocrates. Hope is what comforts, and hope is available even in the most desperate situation. How can we show hope? We can do it by our presence, our touch, and our own assurance that God, the maker of heaven and earth, is in charge.

God is the captain of the healing team. I can close an incision or a wound, but I cannot make the fibrous cells reach across the gap to unite with those on the other side. God programmed that, and he supervises it. God is the one who heals whether I or the sick person believe it or not.

I do believe in him, however, and I have discovered that bringing God into the helping relationship is the most important part of caring for the whole person. In the consulting room, in the operating room, the delivery room, or the emergency room, at the bedside, or in the home, if the Spirit of God and the love of Jesus are alive in me, the God of all comfort will work through me to comfort those in need.

Telling Bad News to Hurting People

Why are we afraid of telling bad news to people who

suffer? In part it is because we fear they will not be able to handle it, and often our fears are justified. We are afraid of adding fear, grief, and depression to an already difficult situation. So we try to hide the bad news by not discussing it. This is a mistake.

We cannot hide bad news from hurting people. They may know the news already, or at least be aware that something bad is happening to them. They will eventually find it out in one way or another and then be angry with us because we have not been up-front with them.

Furthermore, uncertainty is far worse for one's health than bad news. Confusion and hoping for the best while fearing the worst are very difficult for the heart to handle. They add additional anxiety to someone who is already ill. Any attempt at deception is harmful. Sick persons have a remarkable ability to discern insincerity and deception, and this destroys the confidence that is indispensable to the caring relationship.

On the other hand, the truth is therapeutic. Knowledge of the truth, no matter how uncomfortable that truth may be, removes the uncertainty and frees the mind and the emotions to try to cope with the real situation. I cannot count how many times persons with probable terminal illnesses have expressed deep gratitude to us for telling them their true situation. The way in which we tell the bad news, however, is crucial. We must always tell it with hope.

Embracing hope

We cannot convey hope unless we first understand how to face bad news ourselves with courage and hope. During my final year of medical school, I spent four weeks as an extern on a medical ward. Full of enthusiasm, I beheld myself as the champion of life and healing and as the protector from death of all who were sick. In my imagination, I would be fighting against the death angel, denying him access to those for whom I was caring. Boldly I prayed that God would not allow any of those under my care to die during that month. For twenty-seven days, my prayer was answered, and I felt triumphant. My last day on the ward, however, three persons died. I was devastated. I had failed!

My real problem was that I myself could not face the reality of death. I was in denial. For one thing, it represented a failure of my medical capacities. But on a much deeper level, I had not faced up to the possibility of my own death. As a result, during the early years of my practice, a person with an incurable disease was a threat to me. Those who had a malignant tumor, cirrhosis, or progressive heart failure made me uncomfortable. As death approached, I would visit them less often, rationalizing this with the mistaken belief that my time was better spent with those whom I could help to recover. How unwise this was, for those who are approaching their final journey need our presence more than at any other time. I had to face the reality of my own mortality before I could give hope to a dying person. God has taught me much about this in many ways.

How do I as a physician tell a person that he or she has an incurable disease? Is there any way to do this that can somehow give encouragement and hope? The answer is yes, and that is true whether it be multiple sclerosis, leukemia, Lou Gehrig's disease, or even what I consider to be the worst disease in human history: HIV/AIDS. We can offer hope even in desperate situations, and that hope often has remarkable effects.

Hope is physiological, for hope strengthens the emotions, the immune system, and other organs as well. In almost every situation, desperate as it may be, there is at least a ray of hope, and we must emphasize that hope to the fullest extent possible. No physician or other caregiver should ever tell the sick person, "There is no hope. You have only three months to live, and I can do nothing for you." In an African context, that is the worst form of curse, and it is devastating in America and Europe as well.

Brutality has no place in the helping relationship. A sick person comes into my office and sits down. If I look up and say, "I am sorry to tell you this, but you have cancer (or AIDS, or multiple sclerosis)," I am being brutal. The emotional content of these diagnoses (and many others) is enormous, and I do major damage to a person's whole being if I announce bad news in such a harsh way. That person's mind will most likely shut down as anguish, dread, and despair take over, with many negative physiological consequences coming from them.

Such brutality is devastating and we must avoid it entirely. We do so not only by being gentle, but also by doing everything possible to prepare the person psychologically for receiving the bad news. Ideally that preparation begins when we start an investigation that might lead to bad news. If no bad diagnosis is found, we have lost nothing. If we do find bad news, the person is then prepared to receive it with hope.

A living hope
What hope can we offer to a person who has AIDS, or far-advanced cancer, or rapidly progressing cirrhosis of the liver? God has given us a living hope by raising Jesus Christ from death (1 Peter 1:3). If Christ lives within us, death can touch only our physical body, and we will receive a replacement for that. When I arrive in heaven, my physical body will be renewed. It

may look like my earthly body, but the viruses, the rebellious cancer cells, and the fatty plaques plugging my coronary arteries will remain behind. Offering this living hope to those who are dying makes available to them the source of new life. It must never be done, however, by excessive persuasion or attempts at manipulation.

Once hope is restored, persons with heart disease, malignancies, or even AIDS may go into remission and live months and even years beyond that of the expected prognosis.[3] We saw this in chapter 6 where I described Nellie, who lived for ten years with her HIV disease because she determined to care for her children until the oldest two had finished their schooling. Viktor Frankl calls this "logotherapy," which means to find meaning and purpose for life. He survived the horrors of the Holocaust because he had a reason to live.[4]

Preparing people to receive bad news

Adequate psychological and spiritual preparation prior to telling painful news is essential. A sick person is already worried about the illness. Often additional stress may be present from personal problems, conflicts, or painful situations from the past. All of these problems depress the immune system. If we convey bad news abruptly and without preparation, this can devastate an already stressed person and cause severe negative reactions, even suicide.

When I discover that a person for whom I am caring has cancer, HIV, or another serious disease, I refer him or her to one of our pastoral caregivers. The caregivers can help the person deal with the current stress before the additional stress of a difficult diagnosis is added. In this way a person can find adequate strength in soul and spirit to be able to receive the bad news with equanimity.

This takes time. Often our staff will spend hours with a person in a series of dialogues. The pastor listens to the whole story. She or he will usually explain who Christ is and how a commitment to Christ can bring new life and hope into the situation. If the person is interested, the pastor will invite him or her to enter into a relationship of trust in God through Christ. If this step is taken, the person can then bring his or her social, psychological, and spiritual problems to God. Allowing Christ to remove stress and negative emotions and to heal the wounds they have made restores peace and gives courage to the heart. We usually delay the difficult announcement of bad news until the pastor feels the person has gained sufficient inner strength to receive it with courage.

Telling bad news with hope

It is not an easy task to tell a person bad news. It requires time, patience, and a calm spirit. Gentleness is paramount in this process. A slow, gradual approach, using simple, clear language, is usually the best way. It has been our practice for the attending physician and the pastor to meet together with the sick person to reveal the bad news. Since we are dealing with a medical diagnosis, the physician takes the initiative.

I will describe here how, as a team, we explain the diagnosis to a person who has AIDS. I follow a similar approach when dealing with cancer or another potentially fatal disease. It is important to remember, however, that whatever the disease may be, each person is different. Following a set pattern or an impersonal routine has no part in this process.

To put the sick person at ease, I ask about any changes that may have occurred since we began caring for him or her—signs of improvement, or new problems. I then continue as follows. "I want to explain to you the results of our examinations so that you will know what your situation is. You have a right to know this because, with this knowledge, you will know better how to cope with your illness. We can then work together with you to help you fight the disease and find ways to strengthen your health. [I am already trying to convey hope.]

"Our laboratory tests show that you have an infection caused by a virus. Unfortunately, antibiotics do not work against viruses, so we have no specific cure for your infection. Nevertheless, there are things you can do to cope with this infection, and we will discuss these with you in a moment. [Here I am emphasizing that certain things can be done.] The infection you have is quite common and many people suffer from it. The virus I am talking about is the one that causes AIDS. In other words, we have found that you have AIDS."

At this point I pause briefly to see if there is an immediate reaction, or any questions. If so, the pastor and I will deal with this together. We then talk to the person about the future, and give recommendations about various ways to protect and strengthen his or her health—good nutrition, protection against the common diseases, coming quickly for treatment when another infection does occur.

We discuss changes that may be necessary in behavior or living conditions. We use dialogue and adapt what we recommend to the person's particular situation. We review the implications of the illness on his or her future and talk about how to make maximum use of the remaining months or years.

We try to help the sick person set goals for the coming days. We encourage him or her to come back regularly for visits and give assurance that we will always be available for help and support.

HIV infection is notorious for causing severe depression and even suicide. We have informed more than one thousand persons of their disease, and we have yet to encounter a serious reaction of depression. We have never observed even a threat of suicide. Grief is frequent and this is normal. Questions and concerns are many, and we discuss them together.

Throughout the whole process we try to convey hope and the fact that we will continue to accompany the sick person throughout the illness. The journey may be difficult, but we will be there to help them, to give whatever treatment is possible, to give comfort, to pray, and to hold their hand. We need to remember that, as Christian caregivers, we are the physical embodiment of Jesus Christ who promised never to leave us or forsake us.

God, Medicine, and Miracles

Caring for the whole person is the exciting frontier of medicine today. Bringing together faith in Christ and the full range of health sciences opens possibilities for many wonderful healings to occur that might not otherwise take place. It will also open the door wider for God to do more wonders in our midst as we see how God, medicine, and miracles fit together.

Notes

Chapter Two: Words That Heal

1. Matthew 13:14-15; Mark 4:12; Luke 8:10; John 12:40; Acts 28:26-27.
2. Bernard Lown, introduction to *The Healing Heart*, by Norman Cousins (New York: Norton, 1983) 16.
3. Lown, 13-15.

Chapter Three: God Made Us Whole

1. "Put on the new self which God, its Creator, is constantly renewing in his own image, in order to bring you to a full knowledge of himself" (Colossians 3:10).

Chapter Four: The Chemistry of Emotions

1. Hans Selye, *The Stress of Life* (New York: McGraw-Hill, 1984).
2. Norman Cousins, *Anatomy of an Illness as Perceived by the Patient* (New York: Norton, 1979).
3. The following two books discuss the complex elements of the immune system:

Paul Pearsall, *Superimmunity: Master Your Emotions and Improve Your Health* (New York: Fawcett, 1987). In the first three chapters of this book, Dr. Pearsall describes how certain organs and different types of white blood cells interact to protect our health and to cope with many diseases.

Norman Cousins, *Head First: The Biology of Hope and the Healing Power of the Human Spirit* (New York: Penguin, 1989). In chapter

3, Cousins discusses how biochemicals produced by the brain strengthen our immune system and combat infections and malignancies.

4. Pearsall 18.

5. For a detailed and well-documented discussion of the relationship between stress and health, see Bruce S. McEwen, "Protective and Damaging Effects of Stress Mediators," *New England Journal of Medicine* 338, no. 3 (15 January 1998): 171–79.

Chapter Five: The Architecture of the Heart

1. Paul Tournier, *The Healing of Persons* (New York: Harper and Row, 1965) xii.

Chapter Six: What's Sin Got to Do with It?

1. Karl A. Menninger, *Whatever Happened to Sin?* (New York: Hawthorne Books, 1973).

2. St. Augustine, *Confessions.*

Chapter Seven: What's Jesus Got to Do with It?

1. "We are healed by the punishment he suffered, made whole by the blows he received" (Isaiah 53:5).

2. "It is by his wounds that you have been healed" (1 Peter 2:24).

3. David A. Seamands, *Healing for Damaged Emotions* (Colorado Springs: Chariot Victor, 1991).

4. Frank Morison, in his fascinating book *Who Moved the Stone?* (Grand Rapids: Zondervan, 1987), describes from a legal and historical standpoint the overwhelming evidence for the bodily resurrection of Jesus Christ on Easter morning.

Chapter Eight: Heart Cleaning

1. For a helpful discussion of the integration of faith and psychological technique, see Dr. Paul Tournier, *The Person Reborn* (London: SCM Press, 1966).

2. Dr. Lawrence Crabb, in his book *Understanding People: Deep Longings for Relationship* (Grand Rapids: Zondervan, 1987), has an excellent discussion of the relationship between biblical counseling and psychological techniques.

3. David Belgum, *Guilt: Where Psychology and Religion Meet* (New York: Prentice-Hall, 1963) 54.

4. Catherine Marshall has a wonderful discussion of the forgiveness of others in her book, *Something More* (New York: McGraw-Hill, 1974), in the chapter entitled "The Aughts Against the Anys."

Lewis Smedes's book, *Forgive and Forget: Healing the Hurts We Don't Deserve* (San Francisco: Harper and Row, 1984), is also a very sharp and comprehesive study of forgiveness.

5. Mrs. William J. Cox, Tulsa, Oklahoma, used by permission.

Chapter Nine: Free to Be Healthy

1. Dr. Jeffrey Satinover, a psychiatrist in New England, has written a detailed study on compulsive behavior entitled *Homosexuality and the Politics of Truth* (Grand Rapids: Baker, 1996). See pages 130–145.

2. The following books offer effective help for dealing with depression:

William Backus, with Marie Chapian, *Telling Yourself the Truth* (Minneapolis: Bethany House, 1980).

William Backus, *Learning to Tell Myself the Truth* (Minneapolis: Bethany House, 1988).

David A. Seamands, "Dealing with Depression" in *Healing for Damaged Emotions* (Colorado Springs: Chariot Victor, 1991).

Chapter Eleven: Illness: Tragedy or Challenge?

1. Bernie Siegel, *Love, Medicine, and Miracles* (New York: Harper and Row, 1986).

2. Dr. Bill Little, a clinical psychologist and former team psychologist for the St. Louis Cardinals and the Seattle Mariners, has written a helpful book on ways to take a proactive approach to health: *Eight Ways to Take an Active Role in Your Health* (Wheaton, Illinois: Harold Shaw, 1995).

3. Dr. Dale Matthews has written a helpful book called *The Faith Factor* (New York: Viking, 1998). He synthesizes research done in many medical centers on the role of prayer and faith in health and healing. For an annotated, extensive bibliography of articles on the relationship between faith and health, see *Faith Factor*, Volumes I–IV, NIHR Products, 6110 Executive Blvd, #908, Rockville, MD 20852

4. Taylor Caldwell has written two insightful books of fiction about prayer: *The Listener* (Garden City, N.Y.: Doubleday, 1960) and *No One Hears but Him* (Garden City, N.Y.: Doubleday, 1966). These books acknowledge Christ as the unseen listener who not only listens but often replies to the depths of our heart as we talk to him.

Chapter Twelve: Finding Hope in Dark Places

1. Viktor Frankl, *Man's Search for Meaning* (New York: Washington Square, 1959) 104.

Appendix: The Healing Team

1. Leo Tolstoy's telling story, *The Death of Ivan Illyich* (New York: Penguin, 1960), tells a penetrating and disturbing story of what happens to a dying person who does not have quality relationships or anyone to listen to him. It is thoughtful reading for all physicians and other professional caregivers.

2. Dr. Paul Tournier discusses this in his book, *A Listening Ear* (Minneapolis: Augsburg, 1984)

3. Bernie Siegel and Norman Cousins describe the potent physical effects that often follow when persons with a malignant disease find new hope. Siegel's books include *Love, Medicine, and Miracles* (New York: Harper and Row, 1986) and *Peace, Love, and Healing* (New York: Harper Perennial, 1989). Cousins's books include *Head First* (New York: Penguin, 1989).

4. Viktor E. Frankl, *Man's Search for Meaning* (New York: Washington Square, 1959) 104.

Further Reading

The following books, written from various perspectives, provide more detailed insights into some of the subjects discussed in this book.

Backus, William. *The Good News About Worry*. Minneapolis: Bethany House, 1991. How to apply the truth of the gospel to the problems of worry, fear, and anxiety.

____. *The Healing Power of a Christian Mind*. Minneapolis: Bethany House, 1996. How biblical truth promotes health not only of the mind but also of the body.

____. *Telling Each Other the Truth*. Minneapolis: Bethany House, 1991. How the truth can help heal relationships between people.

____. *Telling the Truth to Troubled People*. Minneapolis: Bethany House, 1985. Basic elements of counseling, and how to approach common disorders.

Backus, William, and Marie Chapian. *Telling Yourself the Truth*. Minneapolis: Bethany House, 1980. How biblical truth has the power to bring healing to people.

Benson, Herbert, with Miriam Z. Klipper. *The Relaxation Response*. New York: Avon, 1976. Dr. Benson, a cardiologist, demonstrates from a clinical and research standpoint the connection between the emotions and the circulatory system. Also by Benson (with Marg Stark): *Timeless Healing: The Power and Biology of Belief*. New York: Scribner's, 1996.

Brand, Paul, with Philip Yancey. *Fearfully and Wonderfully Made*. Grand Rapids, Mich.: Zondervan, 1980; and *In His Image*. Grand Rapids, Mich.: Zondervan, 1984. Dr. Brand, a renowned surgeon and specialist in leprosy, writes about the wholeness of human life, using various organs and organ systems as analogies. He has deep insights into the human spirit and how God has created us as whole persons in his image.

Cannon, Walter B. *The Wisdom of the Body*. New York: Norton, 1963. Dr. Cannon discusses how the various organs and organ systems of the body work together in a dynamic equilibrium and how they respond together to the needs of the body.

Cousins, Norman. *Anatomy of an Illness as Perceived by the Patient*. New York: Norton, 1979. Contains a graphic description with many comments of the author's recovery from a potentially fatal illness as he mobilized his thoughts, emotions, and beliefs to improve his immune system. This account deeply impressed the medical community and helped to raise awareness of the interconnectedness of emotions and the body.

——. *Head First*. New York: Penguin, 1989. Cousins writes of his experience in university and research hospitals in California as he helped persons suffering from serious illnesses mobilize their hope. He shows how hope has physiological effects and can lead to improvements in health and the strengthening of recuperative powers.

——. *The Healing Heart*. New York: Norton, 1983. Cousins describes his recovery from a severe heart attack and the role that stress plays in heart disease.

Crabb, Larry. *Understanding People*. Grand Rapids, Mich.: Zondervan, 1987. Dr. Crabb describes how an understanding of people is essential for the helping relationship.

Frankl, Viktor. *Man's Search for Meaning*. New York: Simon and Schuster, 1984. Dr. Frankl, an eminent psychiatrist and a survivor of the Holocaust, shows how an understanding of a higher meaning for life can strengthen health and enable a person to cope with immense difficulties.

Matthews, Dale, with Connie Clark. *The Faith Factor*. New York: Viking, 1998. Dr. Matthews is an associate professor of medicine at Georgetown University in Washington. He draws on more than 400 articles in current medical literature to show how prayer and participation in religious activities promotes health and facilitates healing from serious illness. He believes that the lack of faith and religious experience is a risk factor to health.

Pearsall, Paul. *Superimmunity: Master Your Emotions and Improve Your Health*. New York: Fawcett, 1987. Writing for the layperson, Dr. Pearsall, a clinical psychologist, shows how our emotions are directly related to our health and to our susceptibility to many diseases.

Satinover, Jeffrey. *Homosexuality and the Politics of Truth*. Grand Rapids, Mich.: Baker, 1996. Dr. Satinover, a psychiatrist, gives a clear description of how the chemistry of the emotions relates to behavior, compulsive behavior patterns, and addictions. He also shows how a strong religious experience can bring radical changes to behavior patterns.

Seamands, David A. *Healing for Damaged Emotions*. Colorado Springs: Chariot Victor, 1981. Seamands, a pastoral counselor, shows how our emotions become damaged through life experiences and how healing of these emotions can occur through a realistic and biblical approach.

Selye, Hans. *The Stress of Life*. New York: McGraw-Hill, 1956. Dr. Selye has done basic research on the effects of short-term and long-term stress on the body. He demonstrated in a scientifically rigorous manner the deleterious effects on many physical processes of chronic stress. This book, written in nontechnical language, is a classic.

Siegel, Bernie S. *Love, Medicine, and Miracles*. New York: Harper and Row, 1986. Bernie Siegel, a cancer surgeon, discovered how emotions and the will to fight against malignant disease play a key role in our response to cancer. Also by Siegel: *Peace, Love, and Healing*. New York: Harper Perennial, 1990.

Smedes, Lewis B. *Forgive and Forget: Healing the Hurts We Don't Deserve*. San Francisco: Harper and Row, 1984. Smedes writes about how forgiving others brings healing to damaged feelings and emotions.

Tournier, Paul. *A Doctor's Casebook in the Light of the Bible*. New York: Harper and Row, 1954. Dr. Tournier, a general physician based in Geneva, Switzerland, discovered that life experiences in a sick person are important factors in causing illness. By entering into a helping relationship with sick persons and drawing on the Christian faith and important healing resources in the Bible, Dr. Tournier helped many persons find healing of body, soul, and spirit. His lucid writings have raised awareness of physicians on several continents of the importance of caring for the whole person. Other books by Tournier include *The Meaning of Persons*, New York: Harper and Row, 1957; *The Whole Person in a Broken World*, New York: Harper and Row, 1964; *The Healing of Persons*, New York: Harper and Row, 1965; *The Person Reborn*, London: SCM Press, 1967; *A Listening Ear*, Minneapolis: Augsburg, 1987.

About the Author

A graduate of Colgate University, the University of Rochester, and Johns Hopkins University, Dr. Daniel E. Fountain served as a medical missionary in the Congo for thirty-five years with the American Baptist Board of International Ministries. During that time, he was the director of health services of the Baptist Church of Western Congo and the director of Vanga Evangelical Hospital in the Democratic Republic of Congo (formerly Zaire). Dr. Fountain is the founder and former director of several health programs in Africa, including a health care training institute and a rural health care network. A recognized authority on the treatment of persons with AIDS, Dr. Fountain is the recipient of numerous awards for community health service. In 1984, he and Rev. Felicity Matala established an integrated medical-pastoral care ministry in the Vanga Hospital for the healing of the whole person. He directed the ministry until 1996.

Dr. Fountain currently serves on the faculty of the Christian Medical and Dental Society Continuing Medical Education Program and is an international health consultant for MAP International. He is the author of numerous articles and books. His previous books include *Primary Diagnosis and Treatment; Let's Build Our Lives;* and *Health, the Bible and the Church.* Dr. Fountain teaches internationally about the importance of caring for the whole person. A gardener and a musician, he makes his home in Michigan with his wife, Miriam. The couple have three grown children and six grandchildren.